Pompoir

D.A. Da Costa Intimacy Enhancement Trainer

Copyright © 2010 D.A. Da Costa Intimacy Enhancement Trainer.

ISBN- 13: 978-1478311508

ISBN- 10: 1478311509

Library of Congress Cataloging-in-Publication Data

D.A. Da Costa Intimacy Trainer - Pompoir A Manual Of Ancient Arts to Train And Control The Pelvic Floor.

DISCLAIMER!

This book is intended for mature, adult audiences. All readers or viewers must be 18 years or older, by looking at or reading this book you verify you are at least 18 years or older.

We are not medical doctors or licensed to practice psychology. Pompoir A Manual to Train and Control the Pelvic Floor is not intended to substitute for psychological counseling, or medical treatment for any condition. This book is simply a philosophy of exercise based on ancient techniques.

The use of information on this book is the responsibility of the reader. Should you decide to act on the suggestion of this book and its exercises, you wave all the rights to any type of lawsuit against the author of this book.

DEDICATION

To all the women of the Da Costa and Alves families for being such an inspiration of passionate femininity and strength. This book is a legacy for our little Princesses Raquel, Arianyy, Maria Eduarda , Emily , Priscila B. Oliveira and my eternal angel Elza Suzana da Costa Alves.

TABLE OF CONTENTS

Chapter 1

The Art Of Pompoir

Pompoir…….…...…………………………………......….….02

The Ancient Herstory of Pompoir……….…......……….03

Pompoir Skills ……………………………….…….…..05

Pompoir vs. Kegel………………………….…...07

The PC Muscles …………………………….……09

Chapter 2

What Pompoir Can Do For You

Benefits Of Pompoir…………………………………12

Pompoir For Pregnant Women…………………......13

Pompoir for Aging Women …………………..…….14

Increasing Sexual Desire …………………….....15

Achieving Vaginal Orgasm…………….……..……16

Chapter 3

Pompoir Basics

What You Need for Pompoir.............................18

Sex Toys And Pompoir....................................19

Accessories to Aid Pompoir............................21

The Secrets To Succeed..................................23

Chapter 4

Beginning Your Pompoir Journey

Knowing Your Body.......................................26

Find Your PC Muscles......................... 29

Proper Breathing 30

Learning Your Motions..................... 31

Warm Up and Stretch......................................34

Introduction to Sahajoli..................................36

Pre-Exercise Instructions................................38

Chaper 5

The New "Sahajoli"

Exercise Cycle 1 - Building strength 39

Assignment...44

Exercise Cycle 2 - Getting Tighter.................45

Exercise Cycle 3 - Acquiring Control..............59

Exercise Cycle 4 - Learning Manipulation.........69

Exercise Cycle 5 - Mastering Your Skills 77

Exercise Cycle 6 - Putting All Together.............83

Exercise Cycle 7 - Pompoir With A Partner........87

Chapter 6
Personal Training Program

Your Personal Training Program.....................91

1st Week Program.....................................93

2nd Week Program 94

3rd Week Program.....................................95

4th Week Program 96

5th Week Program 97

6th Week Program.....................................98

7th Week Program 99

8th Week Program…………………………………..100

9th Week Program …………………………………..101

10th Week Program……………………………….. 102/103

11th Week Program……………………………….. 104/105

12th Week Program……………………………… 106

Building Your Exercise Routine …………….. 107

ACKNOWLEDGMENTS

Writing this book was a bit like gathering some raw materials and through an extensive refining process, shaping them into a finally tuned, high performance machine – it takes a great team of skilled and dedicated people to see a concept, and then turn it into reality. I've been gifted with this group of amazing people working with me on Pompoir, and I appreciate each person who gas contributed.

I like to thank my grandmother Dona Maria Jose, who taught me never to quit, my mother to push me further, my sister Debora Zani for being my steady ground, and my cousin Luciane and Luana whom always says it will work it out! I just can't thank enough the matriarchs and my guiding light – Clarisse Ayres , Esmeralda Alves and Ana Maria Alves.

I thank God to bless me with such wonderful family and all the great, unique people that I have met in my life.

I want to thank all the ladies who come to my workshops, thank you so much for the gift of your precious time.

To my dad, I know you would be proud. I love you!

Every success story has a beginning

Throughout my years as a Sexuality Counselor and as an Intimacy Enhancement Trainer, I have heard many of the same worries from women of all body types, ages, and ethnicities: "I feel like my vagina is too large and I often do not feel much sensation during intercourse." The statement is usually accompanied by feelings of confusion and great sexual frustration. With no understanding, women see no resolution in sight and often develop an aversion to intercourse altogether, choosing abstinence over disappointment until finally they reach out for help.

In a majority of cases, these women have never experienced an orgasm through penetration. The temporary solution of using various sensation-enhancing creams is not enticing to many women, and reconstructive surgery is usually not a desired option.

It took a little time, but I delved into the study of Tantric yoga and Tao, amassing a significant amount of research to find answers that will give these women the means to achieve the most satisfactory and rewarding sex lives possible. The results have been very rewarding.

From dozens of different possibilities, I selected individual techniques and combined them into a complete routine. The result is a series of seven fantastic pelvic exercises, that I like to call the "New Sahajoli," because they lead to the mastering of Pompoir skills in the same reported amount of time, that reportedly would take a Ancient Hindu Devadassi.

The set of exercises focuses solely on the manipulation of the PC muscles towards fitness, naturally promoting sexual confidence, improving sexual health and enhancing sexual satisfaction.

This book will give you a complete routine from the basic foundation to mastering all your Pompoir skills. With this set of basic Sahajoli exercises you can build your own stairway to the Mastery of Pompoir.

Before you start any exercise, you need to know exactly which Muscle you are exercising. If you do not know where the muscle is, just follow the tips on page 29 "How to find you PC Muscles."

You should follow the Warm Up and Stretch guide from page 34.

We also include a Personal Training Program with 3 months of Weekly exercises. This ensures that you will build your skill with the right foundation. This fun and easy-to-follow program also includes a daily "Assignment" starting on your second week of training. You can find your assignment on page 44.

Your personal training program will ask you to perform an exercise cycle and a sequence corresponding to that cycle. Sequences can vary from I to IX steps.

Example: *Exercise cycle 1 on page 39, will have 4 sequences, just observe sequence I to IV.*

Your Personal Training Program will give weekly calendars of exercise as a reference, so you are sure to

progress on your Pompoir Skills. Your Personal Training
starts on page 91.

INTRODUCTION TO POMPOIR

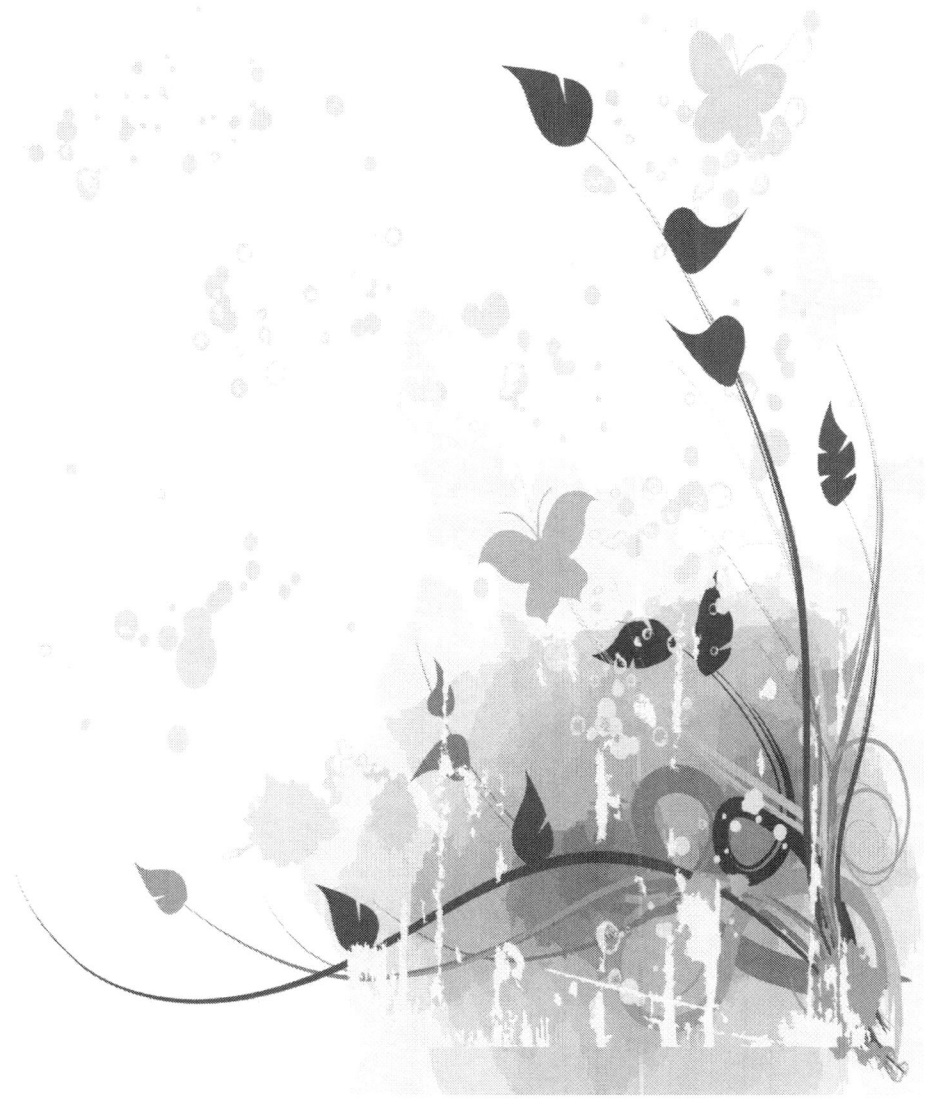

WHAT IS POMPOIR?

Pompoir is referred to as a sexual art and technique that requires extensive training and control of the vaginal or PC muscles. Pompoir Originates from the ancient tradition of Hindu Devadassi. **Pompoir** skills are achievable by a training technique called sahajoli. Throughout the times, Pompoir has also been referenced in different practices, such as "holding firm" in Taoism, "the velvet grip"or kabazza in the Arabic language. The word kabazza translates as 'holder', and the sensation can be likened to 'milking'. The kabazza name is also adopted by South Asia and indicates the female ability to use only the abdominal and vaginal muscles contractions to stimulate the penis of the male partner, while remaining totally passive. The art and sexual technique of Pompoir from ancient times travels to the early followers of the Tantra, Tao and Kama Sutra, and is recognized by sexologists to provide a variety of health benefits. The learning and development of such technique is reported to take months, sometimes years before proficiency is achievable.

THE ANCIENT HERSTORY OF POMPOIR

Historically, in the Far East, sexual knowledge was valued as an important part of a person's cultural education. Societies understood how important the joyful union of the sexes was for male-female relationships and marriage. Over thousands of years, sexual knowledge was refined and passed down to each succeeding generation. Some of this knowledge was eventually recorded in works such as the *Karma Sutra*, the *Ananga Ranga*, and the *Tao Te Ching*.

A woman trained in the Pompoir art masters control of her pubococcygeus muscle (PC) and other pelvic floor muscles, giving her the ability to clutch or grip a penis with her vagina and rhythmically squeeze it as if milking it. The *Ananga Ranga* compares this to the motion of a hand milking a cow. This practice first became known in the West through Sir Richard Burton's translation of *The Kama Sutra of Vatsyayana*, where an account was given describing how a wife pleases her husband and herself using vaginal constrictions.

Women skilled in the art of Pompoir were traditionally trained on sahajoli techniques by an already-initiated older female. Sometimes, the student's mothers or grandmothers were assistants in the role of shakii or sexual initiation to expedite the learning of vaginal control to girls at the age of puberty.

A mother, aunt or an older experienced woman called the sexual initiatrix was in charge of passing the erotic qualities of the unique feminine essence, as part of the religious practice for the sacred courtesan, "Devadassi" or temple dancers.

The legend of the Devadassi indicates that Hindu Temple dancers had specific ideals of womanhood. They molded their behavior carefully in order to guarantee their mother's love and approval, upon which the women were dependent as they became ready to leave the home. It was believed that to be considered a good woman in India, she must be more than just a perfect daughter. Like the Japanese geishas, they must learn submission, docility and grace in various household tasks that constitute the virtue of womanhood.

Sahajoli is an exercise sequence focused on vaginal muscle control and manipulation. Training often uses dildos or phallic substitutes to facilitate mastery of the technique.

The sacred courtesan Devadassi was highly respected for having acquired the specialized training of sahajoli and achieving the vaginal control needed for Pompoir. Her expertise and experience in the temple operations would have provided her with an understanding on erotic exchange inaccessible to the average woman. The Devadassi is closely associated with vama marga. Vama Marga is the left path of tantra which combines sexual life with yoga practices.

POMPOIR SKILLS - ABILITIES YOU WILL DEVELOP WITH YOUR TRAINING

Suck—You will learn to "suck" the penis like a pacifier through constant vaginal movements (suck, let go, suck, let go, suck, etc.), controlling the speed and duration of each movement. You will learn to suck the full length of your partner's penis or even draw it inside your vagina in three stages (barely inside, inside and maximum penetration), torturing your partner with exquisite, teasing pleasure.

Pulse—You will learn to suck the penis rapidly in strong, intense pulses.

Squeeze—You will learn to squeeze the penis with the rings of vaginal muscle, massaging the whole penis or any portion from head to base.

Expel—You will learn to push the penis out from the vagina with one forceful contraction.

Extruding "like milk a cow" —You will learn to "milk" the penis by combining a muscular squeeze-lock with sucking motions that run up the length of the penis in waves.

Capture—You will learn to pull the penis that is just outside the vagina fully inside using only your vaginal muscles.

Lock—You will learn how to hold the penis inside using the strength of the vaginal rings.

Twist—You will learn to make side-to-side movements using the center muscles of your vagina.

HOW POMPOIR DIFFERS FROM KEGEL

Overview of Kegel

Dr Arnold H. Kegel, MD, gynecologist (1894 -1981) invented the Kegel exercises in order to treat his patients that have lack of bladder control.

Pelvic muscle exercises, also known as Kegel, had the objective of treating urinary incontinence. When performed correctly, these exercises help to strengthen the muscles at your bladder outlet. Through regular exercise you can build strength and endurance to help improve, regain, or maintain bladder and bowel control.

Kegel will help you build strong PC muscles while Pompoir will help you build strong, tighter Muscles, and give you the ability to control and manipulate

How to do Kegel Exercises

The Kegel consist on sustained and short contraction of the PC muscle alternating with equal periods of relaxation. If correctly done, Kegel provide many benefits such as the prevention of urinary and fecal incontinence, prevention of a prolapsed bladder, and preparation of women for childbirth. Improved muscle tone and increased sexual fulfillment are also recognized benefits.

Pompoir provides all the benefits of Kegel exercises, and carries them further. The primary advantage of Pompoir is that once mastered, the woman will be able to increase the sexual pleasure of both herself and her partner. It will give you extensive control and manipulation of the pelvic floor.

Overview of Pompoir

Pompoir is a sexual skill where the woman, with her partner and herself remaining still, can induce an orgasm into a man only by moving her vaginal muscles. It takes an extensive set of skills to induce an orgasm in this manner. This, of course, requires intensive training for an extended period of time.

Pompoir skills are acquired through an extensive set of exercises. While the time commitment and intensity is greater than with Kegel, those who master Pompoir are left with stronger muscles them those just practicing Kegel plus the benefit of sexual skills that is not possible to achieve solely through Kegel exercises alone.

Pompoir involves the intense exercise of the vaginal muscles. Its purpose is to acquire the isolated control of the muscles. The skills acquired involve the pushing, pulling, squeezing, twisting and extruding (like milking a cow), of the PC muscles. The principal goal is to give male partners an intense, mind- blowing orgasm.

THE PC MUSCLES

The pubococcygeus muscle, or PC muscle, is a big loop of muscle that looks like a sling and supports the pelvic floor. It encapsulates the internal genitalia, and also supports the uterus. The labia major is part of the ring of muscles directly connected to your PC muscles, and you will be strengthening these muscles as you strengthen your vaginal walls (see the indication on the picture *"pink collared - vagina"*). When you urinate, if you stop and start the stream, you are using the PC muscles. They are also critical to your orgasm, which is why exercising these muscles will enhance your sexual pleasure.

A weak PC muscle can cause urinary and fecal incontinence and sexual problems, such as loss of sensation in the vagina. Obesity, chronic constipation and lower estrogen levels, from menopause, can weaken the muscles. Pregnancy and childbirth can also cause weakness. Pompoir exercises are a great way to strengthen the PC Muscles.

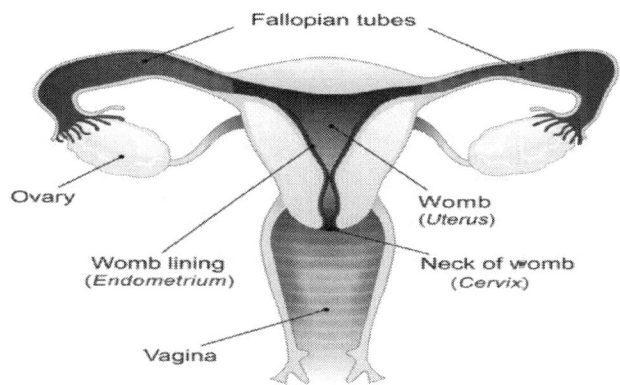

WHAT POMPOIR CAN DO FOR YOU

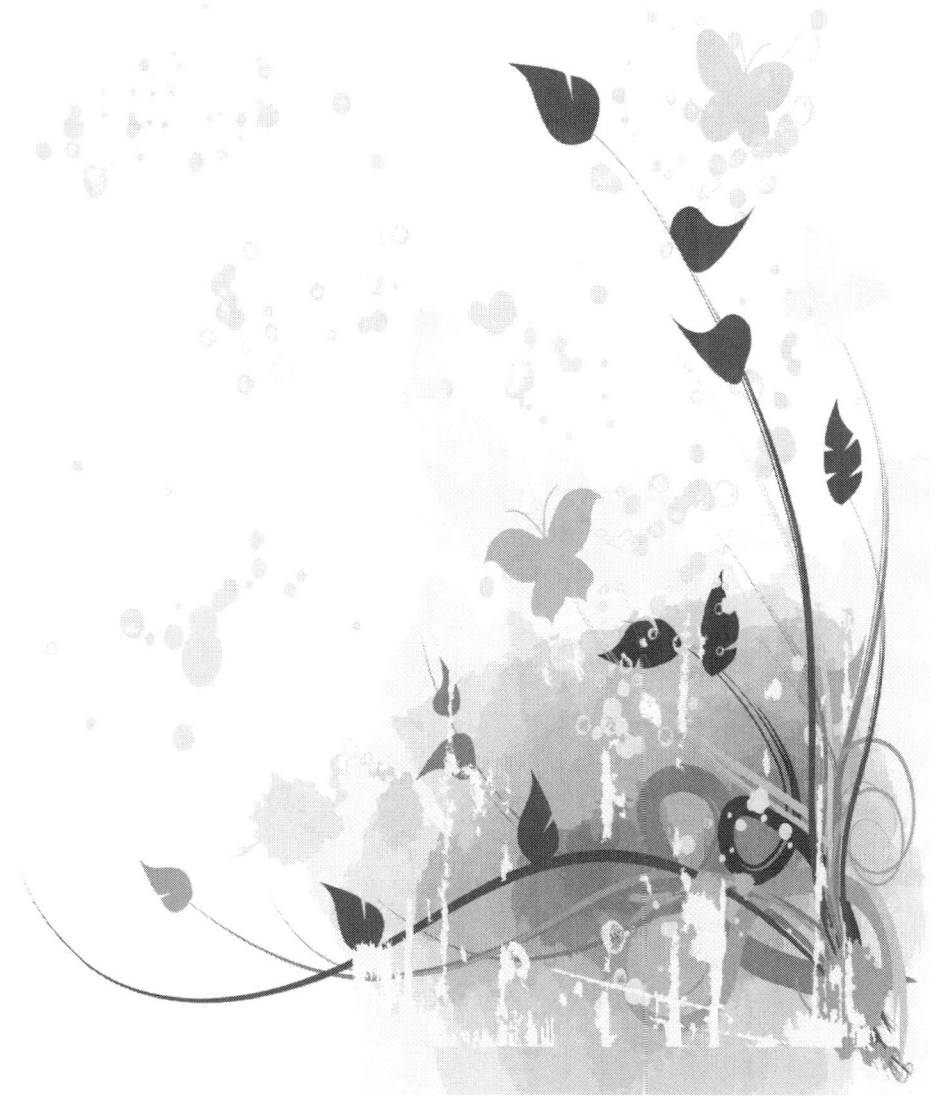

THE BENEFITS OF POMPOIR

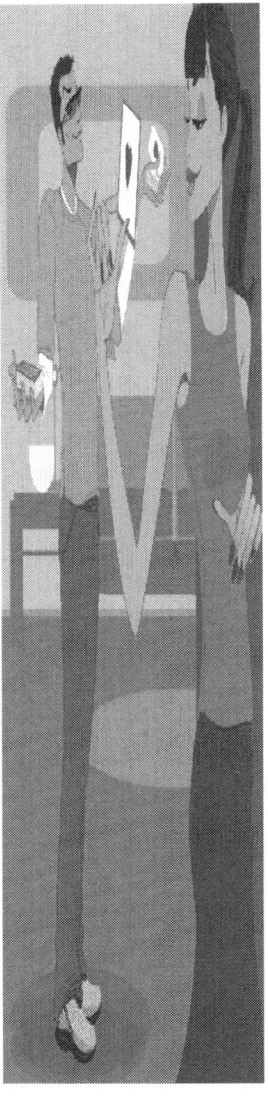

For women

- Awakens sexual responsiveness
- Helps achieve vaginal orgasms
- Helps induce female ejaculation during orgasm
- Helps increase fertility
- Stimulates different levels of sexual enjoyment
- Helps treat and prevent pelvic floor weakness
- Prevents urinary incontinence
- Improves mental well-being
- Stress reliever
- Improves self-esteem
- Boosts sexual confidence

For men

- Longer-lasting intercourse
- Prolonged orgasm
- "Size" doesn't matter for women with healthy and strong PC muscles
- Stimulates different levels of sexual enjoyment
- Boosts sexual confidence

POMPOIR FOR EXPANCTANT MOTHERS

Pompoir exercises have an important role for expectant mothers. These exercises help improve baby delivery by strengthening the muscles of the pelvic floor, which can become weak through pregnancy. During pregnancy a woman's body undergoes significant changes. Exercises can help you relieve the discomfort associated with those changes as well keep you in shape sexually for intercourse after delivery. Pompoir reduces the risk of loss of bladder control during periods of coughing, laughing and sneezing while pregnant. Pelvic exercises are also reported to speed up the healing of a tear or episiotomy (surgical cut made in the perineum to speed up delivery).

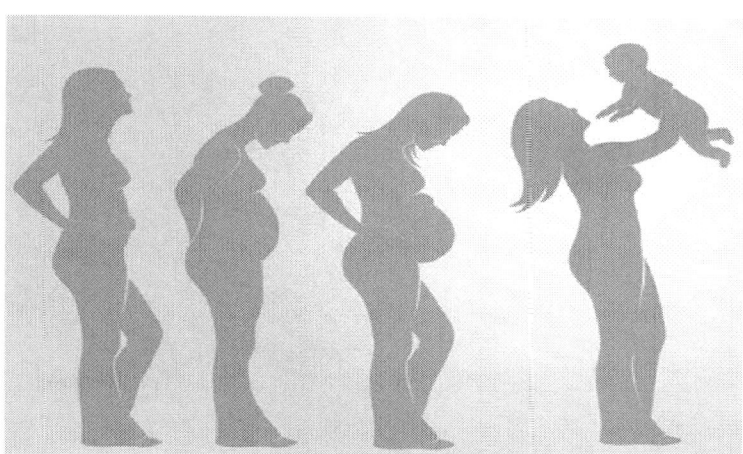

Pompoir exercises empower aging women. Pelvic floor problems due to life events of natural aging, poor diet and hormonal fluctuations such as menopause, can be minimized through Pompoir. During menopause, women can experience a decrease in estrogen which may initiate the thinning and weakening of the pelvic muscles and connective tissues. This makes women more susceptible to decreased tone, elasticity and suppleness in the tissues of the pelvic floor. Strengthening your pelvic floor with Pompoir exercises prior to, and during this time of transition, can lead to a strong healthy core which not only ensures comfort and pleasurable sex throughout the years, but minimizes the chances for urinary and/or stool incontinence later.

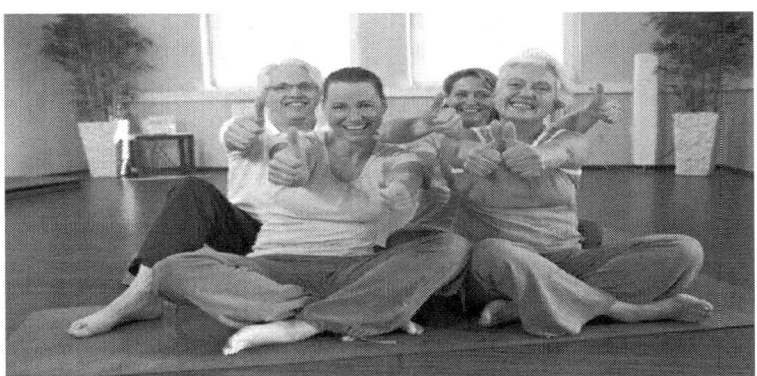

HOW POMPOIR INCREASES SEXUAL DESIRE

Exercise can help bring up your level of sexual desire. While many consider it a fairy tale that exercise improves sex, the types of exercises practiced in Pompoir actually improve the libido and give a spike in sexual desire. Pompoir exercises specifically boost your sexual desire, elevate your self-esteem and improve your vaginal health.

Pompoir cannot improve sexual desire by itself. First, you must have the desire for sex, then Pompoir exercises can put you in the mood. Because Pompoir targets your genital area, some of the building strength exercises can help build the mood and promote sexual activity. The exercises of Pompoir will improve a range of motions, increase flexibility, improve circulation, build desire and give you the confidence to try new things. So, let yourself go and ENJOY!

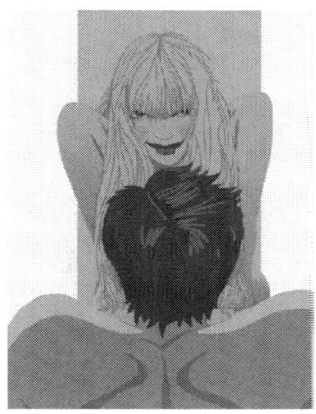

VAGINAL ORGASM WITH POMPOIR

Pompoir exercises tone the vaginal walls and increase the duration and pleasure of orgasms. As you work out regularly to build your Pompoir skills, the exercises will naturally increase blood flow in the vaginal area. The increased blood flow will heighten the sensitivity of the vagina, and will provide tightness of the PC muscles. This tightness will create more friction and give a woman the opportunity to achieve vaginal orgasms. The continuous practice of those exercises will cause the orgasms to be stronger and last longer.

A woman who practices vaginal control can experience greater enjoyment of foreplay and intercourse. She can also stimulate her partner in fabulous new ways! With better stimulation the need for synthetic lubrications is lowered due to the higher sexual response that makes the vagina lubricate itself. The natural body fluids are better and provide a bigger turn on for both partners.

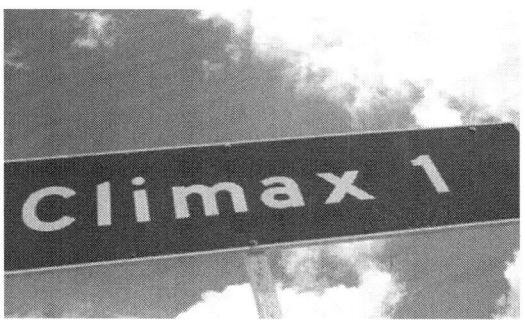

POMPOIR BASICS

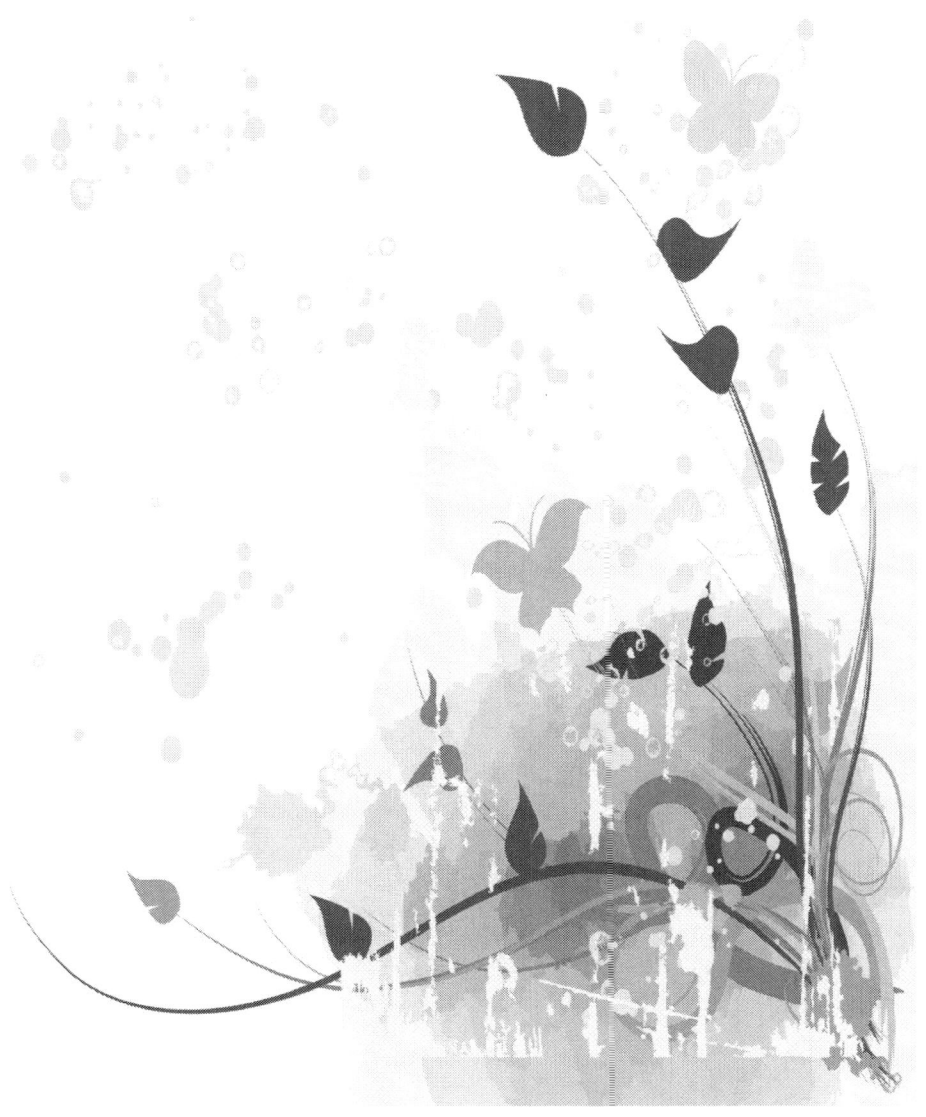

WHAT YOU NEED TO PERFORM POMPOIR

Now that you are familiar with the skills you will achieve and the benefits that will follow, let's take a look at what we need for Pompoir.

- A Private space
- A Clean Towel
- A Mirror
- Pleasure Pods or similar pelvic exercise aids
- Ben Wa Balls or similar pelvic exercise aids
- Cylindrical Vibrator

There are several products available in the marketplace for pelvic exercises. You may already have a few of the aids. We definitely encourage you to try to work with what you already have. Just be sure to note that some commercially available products available for pelvic muscle exercise are too heavy for the beginning of this course. So, you may want to leave the heavier items for a more advanced phase of the exercise regimen, such as Mastering Your Skills, or when you are building your own training program. The ideal practice is to start with something lighter, particularly when it comes to the pods. We are more than happy to give you a list of our favorite items and sizes. They are traditional, easy to find and are perfect for the personal training program we have developed for you.

SEX TOYS TO AID POMPOIR

Wanting to work out and exercise your pelvic muscles is a good idea and a noble goal for women of any legal age; but when it comes to using sex toys as an aid to support the exercises, you might have some concerns. Keep in 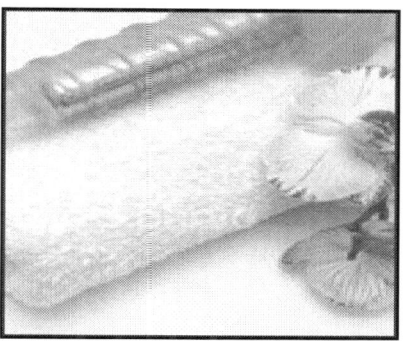 mind that sex toys have been used for centuries to improve sexual performance, especially ben wa balls. The use of the accessories we indicate will help you achieve your goal faster.

Remember, the toys you are buying are meant to aid pelvic exercises. Toy that are suitable for these exercises include pods and ben wa balls. The cylindrical vibrator is an aid you might feel less comfortable with, but it is essential to helping you acquire and master Pompoir skills.

Exercise experts then to state that if you exercise without weights, you will get fit first and have tight and strong muscles later. The opposite is true if you begin with a weight regimen – you will get tight and stronger muscles first, and get fit later. Think of ben wa balls as weights for this exercise program.

The pods are meant to work out the pelvic and vaginal muscles. A great motivational boost on your new exercise journey, all you have to do is wear it, and the work out is done.

The aids are all about taking care of you - your body, your health, your pleasure, your relationship, your womanhood. Healthy pelvic muscles are literally the core of a woman's life-long enjoyment of pleasure, intimacy, and feminine health. Take care of yourself because you deserve to be the best you can be.

ACCESSORIES WE USE TO AID OUR PELVIC FLOOR EXERCISES AND ACHIEVE POMPOIR SKILLS

Pleasure Pods

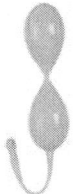

These weighted silicone pods are designed for Pelvic exercises. They are perfect for your training in Pompoir, because they provide maximum results as a part of a daily vaginal exercise program

Ben Wa Balls

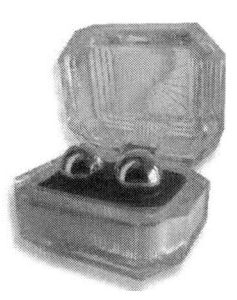

Used since ancient times to tighten pelvic floor muscles. Steel Ben Wa Balls (two Safe Stainless Steel balls – weight of 1.9 oz/Pair) are safe for use and recommended by doctors for performing pelvic exercises such as Pompoir to improve sexual performance and bladder control.

Cylindrical Vibrator

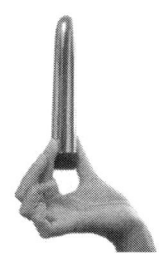

We also recommend that you purchase an old-fashioned vibrator, similar to the one in the photo. The purpose of the cylindrical vibrator is to help you master your skills, especially in manipulating the PC muscles.

IMPORTANT—Never, ever, EVER insert any old substitute—vegetables, kitchen tools, bottles, or any other crazy idea that pops into your head—into your vagina. Not only might this be dangerous and painful, but it might also undo all your fine work toning your vaginal muscles!

IMPORTANT—Do not place accessories inside your vagina when you are having your period.

IMPORTANT— None of the exercises should cause any pain or discomfort. If you feel any of these symptoms, stop immediately. If discomfort continues, see your gynecologist.

IMPORTANT—Do not practice any of your exercises while driving as this will hinder your ability to focus on the road. The idea is to enhance your life!

IMPORTANT—Always clean your accessories (e.g., vibrators, dildos, Ben-wah balls, pleasure pods, etc.) thoroughly after use.

IMPORTANT—Stay healthy. That means not only seeing a gynecologist regularly, but also respecting your body. How long it takes someone to see improvement from these exercises will be dependent on your age, body type, flexibility, diet, lifestyle, and dedication to training. Some of these exercises make take longer than others, but you should see improvement within 6 to 9 months.

THE SECRETS TO SUCCESS IN POMPOIR

Promote Success by protecting your privacy; I advise all of my students to create a safe, emotional space as beginner in the Art of Pompoir. Taking this journey is a very personal decision and you should only share with partners or friends when you feel comfortable doing so. The first few parts of the training are delicate and lead to a feeling of vulnerability. This self -exploration deserves the protection of privacy. The time for sharing your practices with your partner is after you have built up your self-confidence.

Be Persistent. Practice leads to perfection and by consistence practice you will build the skill you need to master the Art of Pompoir. Go slow but keep going, follow the guide lines of the chapters, as you repeat the exercises you see that your awareness of control will grow, as you discover areas of pleasure building your skills at the same time. Don't forget to be kind and encouraging to yourself.

Be Patient. Learning new skills require patience. The first time you explored your sexuality and masturbated, it may have felt good but you probably were unsure exactly how to build this pleasure into an orgasm. The same is true for training your PC muscles and learning the Art of Pompoir. Give it time and allow experience to develop your skill. Enjoy each stage of growth, and don't worry about the "grand finale."

BEGINNING YOUR POMPOIR JORNEY

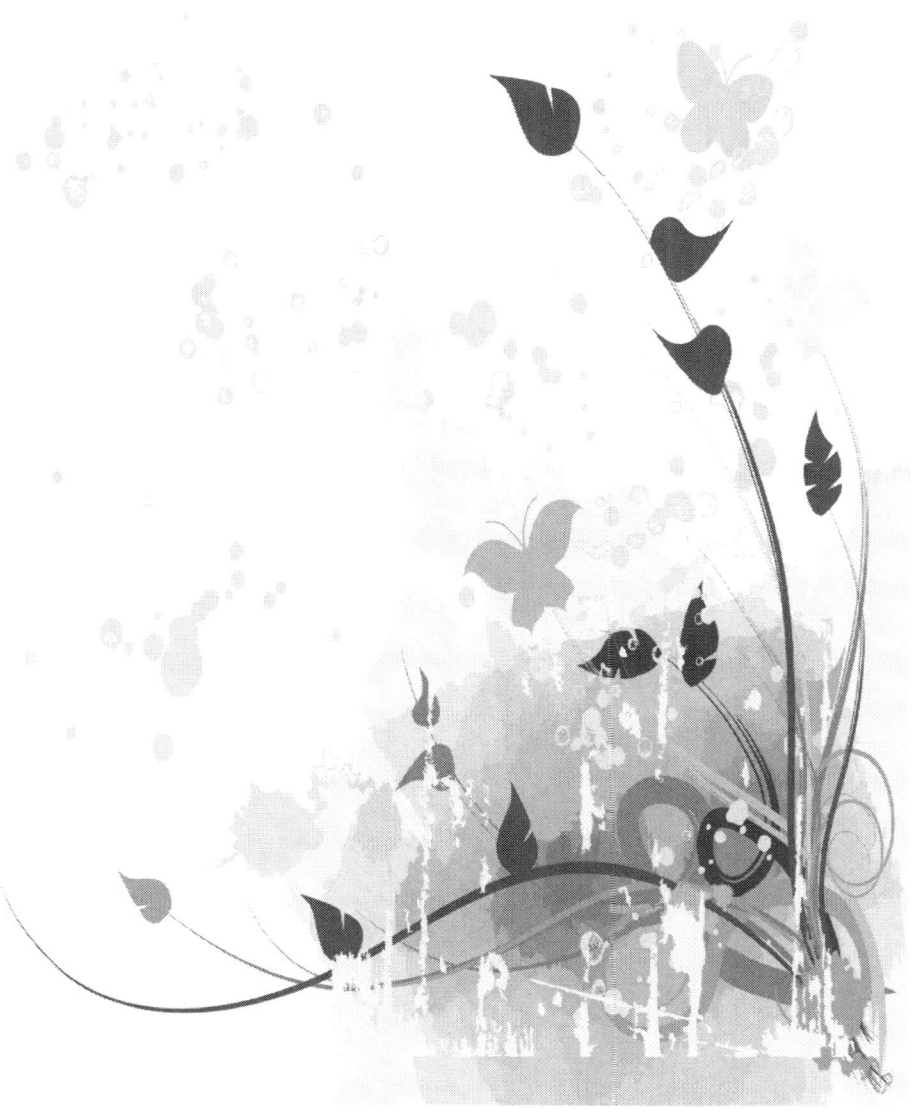

How can you control something that you are not familiar with? You can't. For this reason, there is no better way to begin than getting to know your body, specifically, your genitals. The best way to learn about your body is through self-exploration. For maximum pleasure, you should be relaxed and comfortable.

What you'll need:

A) A mirror

B) Loose or no clothing, at least from the waist down

C) Clean towel

D) A relaxing, safe atmosphere (with no interruptions!)

The Exploration

Once you feel relaxed, sit with your legs open and hold the mirror so you can see your genital area, called the *vulva*. Begin by paying close attention to the entrance of your vagina, exploring the external area first, starting with the *labia majora* ("big lips"), the fleshy flaps of skin on either side of the vulva, and the *labia minora* ("small lips"), the soft, hairless flaps of skin between the labia majora and to either side of the opening to the vagina. Now examine the clitoris. The soft button of flesh, about the size of a pea and located just above the labia, is the *glans clitoris*, the most sensitive area of the female genitalia. This part of the clitoris is tucked under a flap of skin called the clitoral hood, but there is more to this organ; what you cannot see is that the clitoris extends inside the body for several centimeters before branching into two sensitive "legs" spread on either side of the labia minora.

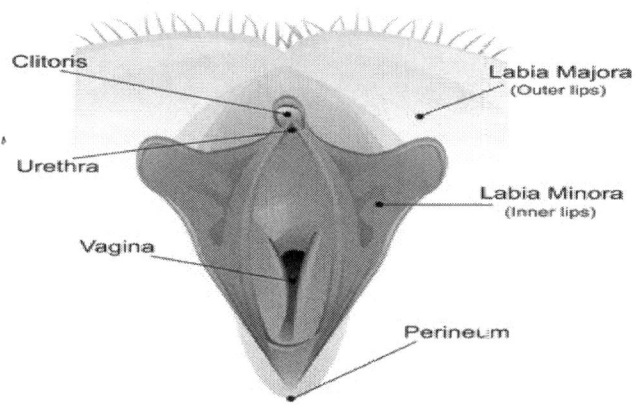

Something else you won't be able to see, but that you will become very familiar with, are the pubococcygeus or PC muscles.

Using your fingers, gently open the entrance to your vagina and try to see as much of it as you can. Insert one of your fingers several centimeters and experiment: using your vaginal muscles, try to see which of these things you can do: squeeze it, suck it in, lock it inside you. See if you can feel the finger rolling toward the side when you move the muscles. Don't worry if you can't do any of these things yet. The exercises will show you how. And if you can already do these things, the exercises will help you become an expert.

HOW TO FIND THE PC MUSCLE

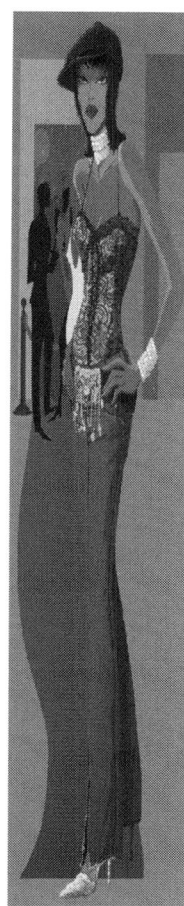

The best way to find your PC Muscle is to stop the flow of urine several times as you sit on the toilet; be sure to keep your legs wide open to avoid the muscles from the buttocks sending confusing signals. Let's break this down into steps that help make it easier to find. When you are ready:

> **Step 1** Sit on the toilet (preferably at the comfort of your home)
> **Step 2** Spread your legs as much as you can.
>
> **Step 3** Try to stop the urinary flow. Do this several times until you can clearly feel the muscle you are using to stop the urinary flow. That muscle is the PC muscle, which is the muscle we will be working.

You can also easily locate your PC muscles when you insert a tampon. The tampon is held by the PC muscles, until removal.

Another way to locate the PC muscles is to ask your doctor for help.

PROPER BREATHING

It's important to stay relaxed during these exercises. One way to help stay relaxed is to maintain proper breathing. Remember to breathe regularly during strength training to establish a rhythm. The biggest problem many have is not that they breathe incorrectly, but rather that they hold their breath. Rhythmic, paced breathing helps to prevent you from getting dizzy.

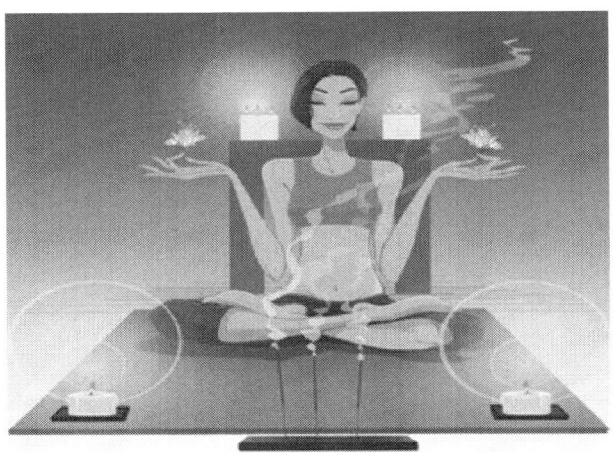

LEARNING THE MOTIONS:
CONTRACT, SQUEEZE, PUSH, PULL AND RELAX

One of the keys to being able to perform Pompoir is being able to recognize the difference of the movements. In the beginning, it is estimated at least 90% of you won't be able to discern the difference between some or even all of the movements. Below, you will find the definitions of the movements. You should take the time to understand the movements such that as you learn how to control your PC muscles, you can begin performing the exercises in the prescribed manner.

Contracting means becoming shorter. To perform the contract motion, you must focus your mind on your vaginal muscles, and imagine that you are closing your vagina.

Squeezing means pressing together. To perform the squeeze motion you want to concentrate your mind on your pelvic floor. Focus on pressing together your vaginal walls. You want to squeeze the pelvic muscle. Make sure to remember to breathe as you perform the squeezing exercise.

Relaxing means to let your PC muscles go back to their normal state. You are not applying any pressure or force.

Pulling To perform a pull motion you need to concentrate your mind on your vaginal muscle. Concentrate on the opening of the vagina. Very slowly, try to close just the entrance of the vaginal area as much as you can, and eventually the vaginal lips will touch each other.

This motion will cause the PC Muscles to pull inside.

Let's try like this: Raise your hand (either one). Make sure your palm is facing down. Now, let's pretend the tips of your fingers are your vaginal entrance. Now bring all the fingers and the thumb together in a way such that only the tips of the fingers are touching each other.

Your vaginal entrance should be touching the lips in a similar manner or you will have "closed doors."

Push

To perform the push motion, you need to concentrate on your vaginal muscle. To better help you, concentrate on the opening of your vaginal entrance. Try to widely open the entrance by pushing your pc muscles. You will experience some of the same sensation as "squeezing."

A simple way to exercise the PC muscle in this fashion is to use this pushing action next time you pee.

We can do another simulation with our hands. Bring your fingers and thumb together in a way that only the tips of the fingers and thumb touch each other. Good! Now, pay attention to the tips of your fingers and thumb as you press down the middle of your fingers onto the thumb. As they touch each other, you will see your fingers open as you press.

Another simulation is:

Put your right hand around your left wrist. Now try to push your left arm outwards with your right arm. Feel how tight they are getting. Now relax your arms and feel the difference. Feel the tension flow out through your fingers and disappear. Focus on the tension as you pull your right arm toward your body and push outward with your left arm.

WARM UP AND STRETCH

One always needs to warm up before any type of exercise. Stretching right after exercise is important to prevent cramping. Pompoir is no different.

Warm Up

In a bed or on the floor, place yourself in a reclined position. Inhale and contract your vaginal muscles vigorously, feeling the pressure inside; exhale and relax the muscles. Contract and relax your pelvic muscles for another 3 sets of 5 times. Rest for 30 seconds or so, then repeat the warm-up for 3 sets of 10 times; rest 30 seconds again, and repeat the warm-up for 3 sets of 15 times. Remember to breathe as instructed earlier: inhale/contract, exhale/relax.

NOTE: Do not rush when executing these movements, it should be calming like when you are doing yoga. Stay relaxed, stay focused.

Stretch

Stretch exercise routine

Phase I: Relax the vaginal muscles by squatting on the floor. Do not contract the vaginal muscles. Now, place the weight of your body on your flexed thighs, count to 21, and enjoy the feeling of relaxation.

Phase II: Lying on your back, place your feet on the wall, contract your vagina, anus, and stomach. Hold the contraction and slowly let your feet climb the wall until your body is elevated in such a way that your weigh rests on your shoulders. Count to 21 while relaxing.

INTRODUCTION TO SAHAJOLI EXERCISE
CYCLES AND SEQUENCES

Sahajoli is the exercise regiment we use to achieve Pompoir skills.

Women must learn to identify and isolate individual muscles. Acquiring the ability to control such actions as pulsing, squeezing, extruding (like milking a cow) and twisting by controlling your pelvic muscles goes a long way to create blissful orgasms for both you and your partner.

Conscientious and continued training in this way is what made the Japanese *Geishas and Thai courtesans so sexually talented; allowing them to propel small objects and extinguish burning candles with their vaginas. While you may not aspire to toss ping-pong balls to an audience using only your vaginal muscles as in the movie Priscilla, Queen of the Desert, heightening sexual pleasure for you and your partner is certainly achievable using this same improved muscle control.*
Enjoy this great genital fitness, as it builds powerful sexual skills.

Ok, is time to grab your accessories and begin our exercise program. Here is what you will need.

* A Private space
* A Clean Towel
* A Mirror

* Pleasure Pods
* Ben Wah Balls
* Cylindrical Vibrator

And yes, NO interruptions!

Pompoir, like any exercise regimen, only yields results after you put in the time and effort. It may, at times, seem silly. You may be asking yourself why you are doing this. But if you exercise to give yourself a great body, why not exercise to give yourself great sex?!!!

Performing Sahajoli - Exercise Cycles and Sequences

We recommend that you read the sequence and cycles before you perform them. Go to your Personal Trainer Guide, go to the week and date you are about to exercise, and read the routine that is asks you to perform. Reading about the exercise in advance gives you a better understanding of the exercise before you perform.

NOTE: None of the exercises are supposed to cause you any pain or discomfort. If you feel any pain, we advise you to stop your exercises immediately and go see a doctor.

NOTE: Perform this exercise slowly. Relax, don't rush. Synchronize your breathing with your actions.

EXERCISE CYCLE 1 – SEQUENCES I TO V.

BUILDING STRENGTH.

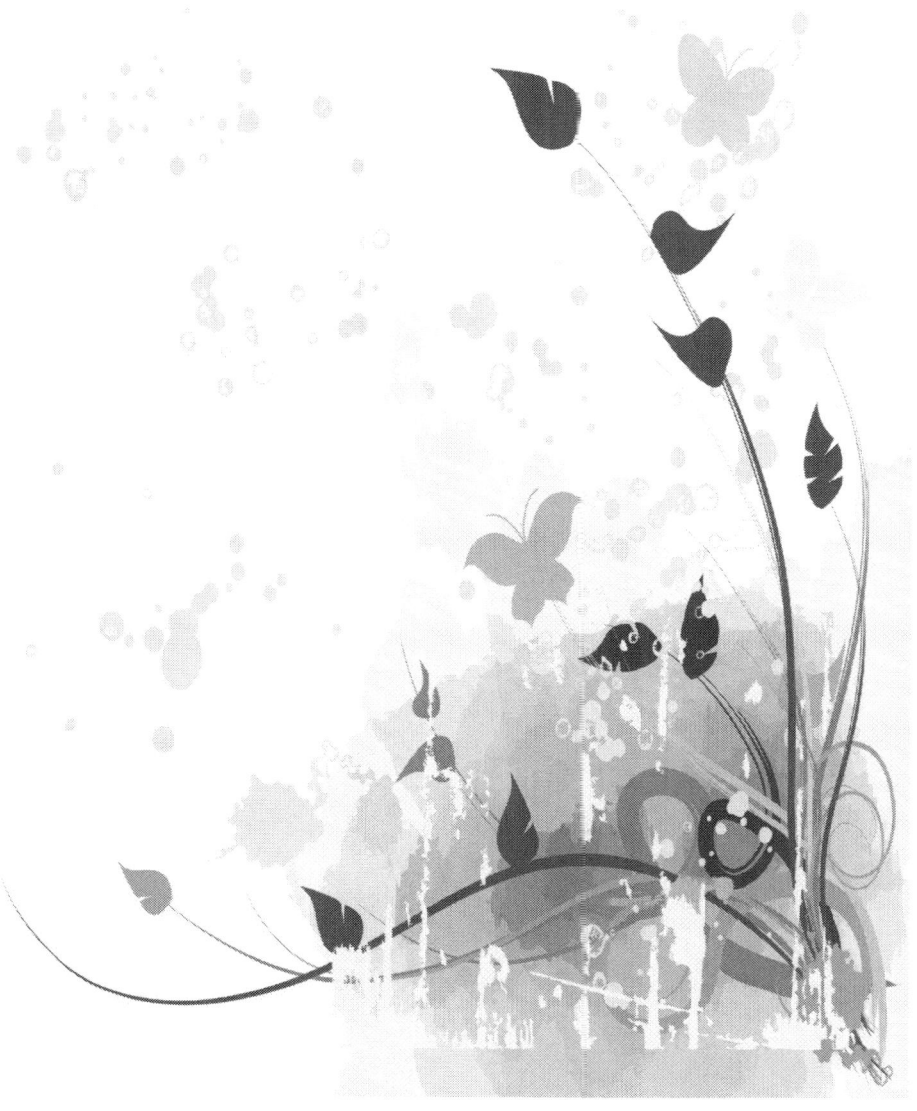

EXERCISE CYCLE 1, SEQUENCE I

Step 1. Sit comfortably in a chair. This helps you resist using your gluteus muscles (buttocks). Don't worry if you find that these muscles still contract somewhat when you tighten your vaginal muscles. This will not ultimately affect your training.

Step 2. Place your hands loosely on your thighs, palms down, keeping your feet on the floor, slightly apart.

Step 3. Inhale. Squeeze your vaginal muscles as though you are holding something inside. Then relax the vaginal muscles as you exhale.

Maintain the position and repeat Step 3 five times. So, you will:

* Inhale and count to five /squeeze / exhale/relax. Repeat this sequence five times.

* Let's keep it up. Repeat the exercise, this time for a count of ten. Inhale and count to ten/squeeze / exhale/relax. Repeat this sequence ten times.

* You are doing well. Let's keep going one more time. This time, count to 15. Inhale, count to 15/squeeze / exhale/relax. Repeat this sequence 15 times.

EXERCISE CYCLE 1, SEQUENCE II

Step 1. Stand with your feet shoulder-width apart and your hands resting comfortably on your hips.

Step 2. Inhale as you squeeze your vaginal muscles as though you are holding something inside. Then, relax the vaginal muscles as you exhale. Now, inhale and contract your vaginal muscles. Then relax the vaginal muscles as you exhale. Be sure to change up the strength and duration of your contractions. Take your time, there is no race to the finish (remember, this is about improving sex)!

Maintain the position and repeat step 2 for a count of five: So you will:

* Inhale and count to five /squeeze / exhale/relax. Inhale, count to five contract / exhale/relax. Repeat this sequence five times.

* Let's keep it up. Repeat the exercise, this time for a count of ten. Inhale and counting to ten /squeeze /exhale/relax. Repeat this sequence ten times.

* You are doing well. Let's keep going one more time. This time, count of 15. Inhale, count to 15 /squeeze / exhale/relax. Repeat this sequence 15 times

EXERCISE CYCLE 1 - SEQUENCE III

Step 1. Still standing with your feet shoulder-width apart and your hands resting comfortably on your hips, ease your pelvis/buttocks backward while inhaling, contracting your vaginal muscles

*Note – Be sure to contract and not squeeze the vaginal muscle.

Step 2. Ease your pelvis/buttocks forward, relaxing the vaginal muscles and exhaling.

Maintain the position and repeat steps 1 and 2 for a count of ten. So, you will:

* Ease your pelvis/buttocks backward while inhaling, contracting the vaginal muscles and counting to ten. Ease your pelvis/buttocks forward, relax the vaginal muscles and exhale. Repeat this sequence five times.

* Let's keep it up. Repeat the exercise, this time for a count of 15. Ease your pelvis/buttocks backward while inhaling, contracting the vaginal muscles and counting to 15. Ease your pelvis/buttocks forward, relax the vaginal muscles and exhale. Repeat this sequence five times.

* You are doing well, let's keep this going one more time. Repeat the exercise, this time for a *count of 20.* Ease your pelvis/buttocks backward while inhaling, contracting the vaginal muscles and counting to 20. Ease your pelvis/ buttocks forward, relax the vaginal muscles and exhale. Repeat this sequence ten times.

EXERCISE CYCLE 1 - SEQUENCE IV

Step 1. Still standing with your feet shoulder-width apart and your hands resting comfortably on your hips, ease your pelvis/buttocks backward.

Step 2. Hold this position for 10 seconds. At the same time, squeeze and release your vaginal muscles rapidly. Inhale as you squeeze and exhale as you release. Take a five second break. Repeat this sequence for 10 minutes

NOTE: Synchronize your breathing with your actions.

NOTE: At the end of this four-phase exercise cycle, you will feel sexually aroused. Not only have you been focusing your mind solely on your erogenous zone, but you have also been performing movements that stimulate the blood flow and excite the nerve endings in the area. Use this exercise any time you want heat up your mood and fire your passion.

Pleasure Pods Work Out!

Step 1 – wash your hands

Step 2 – Take your pods and lube as needed

Step 3- insert the pods inside your vagina

Keep the pods in for 30 minutes as you walk around the house, doing whatever you need to.

Step 4- at the end of 30 minutes, remove the pods and clean thoroughly, store safely for future use.

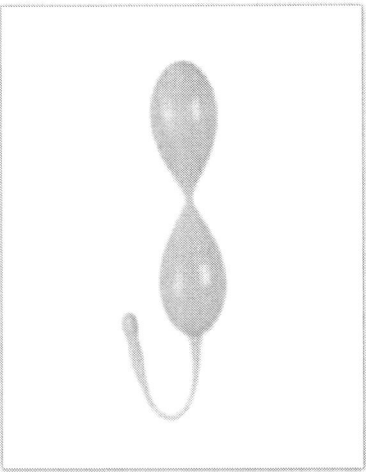

EXERCISE CYCLE 2 – SEQUENCES I TO IX

Getting tighter!

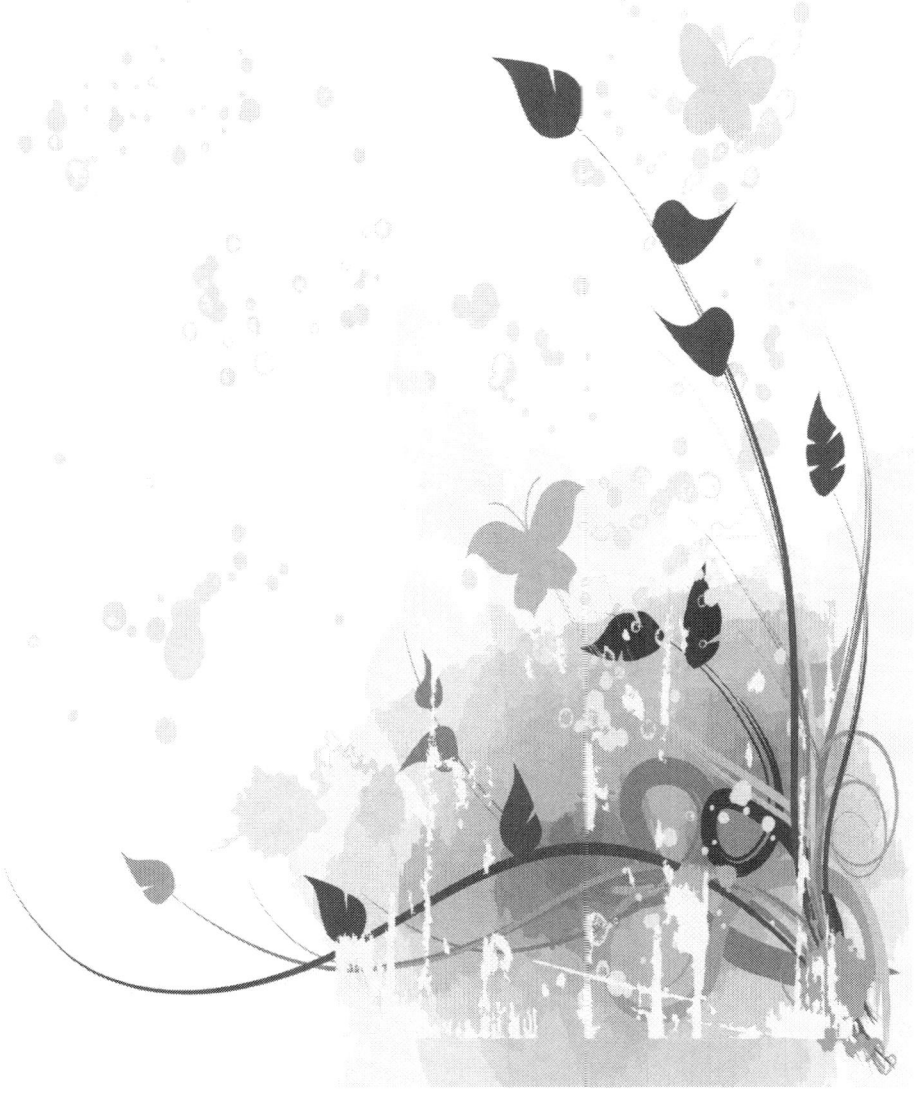

EXERCISE CYCLE 2 – SEQUENCE I

This exercise will help women who experience pain during penetration, generally due to tension or self-consciousness.

Step 1. Stand with your feet slightly more than shoulder-width apart and place your hands comfortably on your hips.

Step 2. Slowly lower your body into a squatting position, keeping your thigh muscles tight while at the same time focusing on keeping your vaginal muscles completely relaxed and open.

Maintain the position and repeat steps 1 and 2 ten times: So you will:

* Inhale/squeeze /stand as you count to ten, exhale/ relax/squat. Repeat this sequence 15 times.

Variation

If you can't squat for any reason here is another variation

Step 1. Sit on a chair with your breast facing the back support of the chair, be sure to keep your back straight. Place your hands comfortably on your knees.

Step 2. Now,

* Inhale/squeeze /stand as you count to ten, exhale/ relax/sit. Repeat this sequence 15 times.

EXERCISE CYCLE 2 - SEQUENCE II

Stand up, legs apart, knees bent slightly, muscles flexed, hands on your waist. The goal of this exercise is to make the pelvis move around, like forming a circle.

Now imagine you breaking the circle in 4 parts: forward, left, backward and right. It's easy! Let's do it together:

Step 1

1. Thrust the pelvic bone forward, pushing your hips to the front. Good now
2. Push the left side of your hips to the left side as far as you can. Keep going
3. Thrust your pubic bone backward , and finally
4. Push the right side of your hips to the right side as far as you can

So, it will be forward, left, backward and right

Step 2

Repeat the following sequence 15 times. . Now let's invert the circle.

1. Thrust the pelvic bone backward, pushing your hips to the back
2. Push the right side of your hips to the right side as far as you can
3. Thrust your pelvic bone forward
4. Push the left side of your hips to the left side as far as you can

Now it is backward, right, forward and left.

Repeat this whole phase six times.

This movement is used in all styles of belly dance and is called "rip circle." It might be a little challenge and tiring in the beginning, but persistence will be very rewarding.

EXERCISE CYCLE 2 – SEQUENCE III

Step 1 – Lay down with your hands alongside your body, with your palms on the floor.

Step 2 - Raise your hips, at same time tightening your gluteus, stomach, and vagina muscles. Hold this position for a count of ten.

Maintain the position and repeat steps 1 and 2 five times. So, you will:

* Raise your hips as described in Step 2. Inhale/ squeeze/ contract & count to six, then exhale/relax. Repeat this sequence five times.

* Let's keep it up. Repeat the exercise, this time repeating the exercise ten times: Raise your hips as described in Step 2. Inhale/ squeeze /contract, count to 6, then exhale/relax. Repeat this sequence 10 times.

EXERCISE CYCLE 2 – SEQUENCE IV

Step 1 - Position yourself on the floor, on your hands and knees. Keep your back straight.

Step 2 - Tighten your vaginal muscles and slowly ease your buttocks back toward your heels until your chest is touching the floor. This exercise not only improves vaginal strength but helps shape the body as well.

To do the push motion, you need to focus your mind. Try to connect the breathing to your physical motions. When you exhale, imagine the air going out of your vagina, so as you exhale you focus on pushing the air out with the vagina in a relaxing motion.

As the exercise becomes easier, increase the number of daily repetitions (up to 30 times per day).

To get started, perform this exercise five times. Inhale/contract/hold count to five. Assume step 1 position exhale/push/relax. Repeat this sequence five times.

* Let's keep this up. Repeat the exercise, this time for a count of ten. Inhale/ contract/hold and count to ten. Assume Step 1 position and exhale/push/relax. Repeat this sequence 10 times.

* You are doing well; let's keep going one more time. Inhale/ contract/hold count to 10. Assume Step 1 position, exhale/push/relax. Repeat this sequence 15 times.

EXERCISE CYCLE 2 – SEQUENCE V

Step 1 - Lie on your back on the floor with your arms relaxed and slightly away from your sides.

Step 2 - Raise your hips, at same time tightening your anus and your vaginal muscles, as hard as you can. Hold this position for a count of 30.

Step 3 - Relax your anus and vagina and lower your hips until your buttocks again touches the floor.

Maintain the position and repeat Steps 2 and 3 ten times.

EXERCISE CYCLE 2 – SEQUENCE VI

Step 1 - Lie on your back on the floor with your arms relaxed and slightly away from your sides, and the soles of both feet flat against a wall at a point about 15 centimeters from the floor.

Step 2 - Tighten your anus, vagina, and stomach muscles; raise your pelvis and buttocks off the floor until your weight rests only on your shoulders and your feet (against the wall). Hold this position.

Step 3 - Relax your muscles and slowly lower your pelvis until your buttocks again touch the floor.

Maintain the position and repeat Step 3 until you count to five: So you will:

* Tighten your anus, vagina, and stomach muscles; raise your pelvis and buttocks off the floor until your weight rests only on your shoulders and your feet (against the wall). Hold this position counting to five/ Relax your muscles and slowly lower your pelvis until your buttocks again touch the floor.

* Let's keep this up. Repeat the exercise, this time for a count of 15. Tighten your anus, vagina, and stomach muscles; raise your pelvis and buttocks off the floor until your weight rests only on your shoulders and your feet (against the wall). Hold this position counting to 15/ relax your muscles and slowly lower your pelvis until your buttocks again touch the floor.

* You are doing well; let's keep going one more time. This time, do a count of 25. Tighten your anus, vagina, and stomach muscles, then raise your pelvis and buttocks off the floor until your weight rests only on your shoulders and your feet (against the wall). Hold this position, count to 25/ relax your muscles and slowly lower your pelvis until your buttocks again touch the floor.

Repeat this sequence ten times.

NOTE: Perform this exercise slowly. There is no hurry. Synchronize your breathing with your actions.

EXERCISE CYCLE 2 – SEQUENCE VII

This exercise will help you contract the vaginal musculature.

Lie on your back with your legs flexed. Place a pillow between your legs, contract the anus and the perineum, count until 20 and relax.

As you feel comfortable, count to higher numbers until you reach 42. Do this exercise from three to five minutes.

EXERCISE CYCLE 2 – SEQUENCE VIII

<u>Step 1</u> - Lie on your back, on the floor. Imagine that you have a balloon in your stomach.

<u>Step 2</u> - Slowly breathe in, filling your lungs and the imaginary balloon with air.

<u>Step 3</u> - Tighten your vaginal, belly and stomach muscles in an undulating sequence, beginning low (with the vaginal muscles) and moving higher (to the stomach muscles).

<u>Step 4</u> – Invert the process as you begin to exhale – start with the stomach and move towards the vagina and then relax your muscles.

Keep focused, and you will be able to perform an undulating sequence.

So you will:

* Slowly breathe in, tighten the vagina, belly and stomach (in a 1,2,3 sequence). Then exhale, slowly inverting the process. Begin with the stomach and work towards the vagina.

Repeat this sequence six times, as it gets easier raise it to eight, then up to ten times.

EXERCISE CYCLE 2 – SEQUENCE IX.

In the same position, contract the vaginal muscles in a fast mode and with intense rhythm. Act as though you are trying to keep up with the panting and breathing. Contract your muscles while inhaling, relaxing while exhaling.

Repeat this movement for about 5 minutes

EXERCISE CYCLE 3 – SEQUENCES I TO V

BEN WA BALLS

ACQUIRING CONTROL!

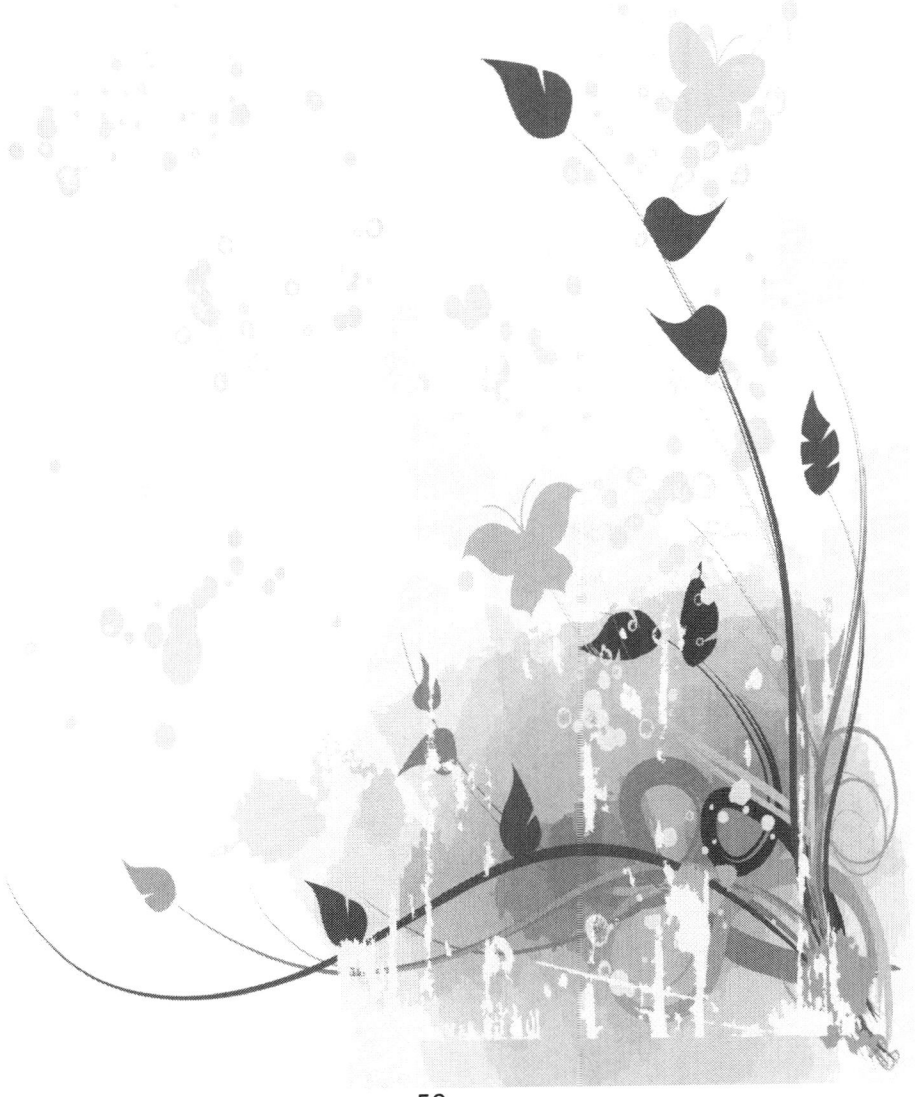

ABOUT BEN WA BALLS

Ben Wa balls have been used for centuries. Taoism and Tantra believe that Ben Wa Balls are helpful tools for Pelvic Exercise control. They are also highly recommended by gynecologists.

Here are some safe tips for the use of Ben Wa Balls.

* Before inserting your Ben Wa Balls, make sure to wash your hands

* Have a towel handy, preferably underneath where you are standing, right between your legs

* Use a lubricator. When you are done, clean the ben wa balls with water and anti-bacterial soap. Dry and place them in a clean, safe place. You may also use toy cleanser.

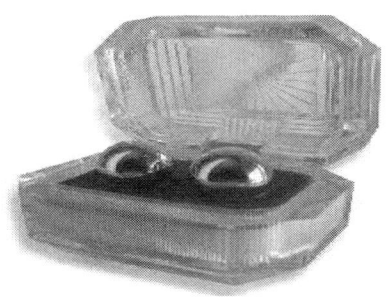

EXERCISE CYCLE 3 - SEQUENCE I

Step 1 - Recline on your bed, or in a cushioned area of the floor, with your legs spread comfortably apart.

Step 2 - Apply gel to the Ben Wa balls and insert one into your vagina.

Step 3 - Place the second Ben Wa ball at the entrance to the vagina. Stand up and try to hold the Ben Wa balls inside of you, by contracting and locking the vaginal muscles.

Maintain the position and normal breathing.

***Step 4** - Stand up and try to keep the Ben Wa Balls inside of you for 5 minutes, then relax (sometimes the balls will come out, and that is ok). Lie down and take the balls out, then clean them. Rest for three minutes.

Note: if the balls come out before the recommended time, don't worry. Take some rest and try the next phase of the exercise. With time, you will be able to keep them inside of you.

* Let's keep it up. Repeat the exercise. Stand up and try to keep the Ben Wa Balls inside of you for 10 minutes, then relax. Lie down and take the balls out and clean them. Rest for three minutes.

* You are doing well, so let's keep going one more time. Stand up and try to keep the Ben Wa Balls inside of you for 15 minutes, then relax. Lie down, take the balls out and clean them. Rest for five minutes before moving on to the next exercise.

EXERCISE CYCLE 3 – SEQUENCE II

We would like to give a note of caution as we enter into that involve reaching deeper into the vagina, You must be especially cautious to stop if you feel any pain or discomfort whatsoever. Take care never to insert anything deep enough that it is forced into the uterus.

Read Steps 1 through 4 before executing.

Step 1 - Recline in your bed, or in a cushioned area of the floor, with your legs spread comfortably apart.

Step 2 - Apply gel to the Ben Wa balls and insert one into your vagina.

Step 3 - Place the second Ben Wa ball at the entrance to the vagina and try to suck it inside. In the beginning, you will probably need to "help" it with you hand, but after regular training you should be able to do this with your vaginal muscles alone.

Step4 - After the 15th effort to suck the second Ben Wa ball into the vagina, we are going to start push out . This sequence will not only greatly strengthen your muscles and control, but it will also be a very pleasurable exercise!

Step 5 - To remove the Ben Wa balls, push them out with your vaginal muscles. You may need to help this effort with your hand.

Repeat the whole sequence two times

ECERCISE CYCLE 3 - SEQUENCE III

Note: Strengthening the muscles is one thing, controlling and manipulating the muscles is another. You've been working hard to acquire these skills, so let's get started

Step 1 - Recline in your bed, or in a cushioned area of the floor, with your legs spread comfortably apart.

Step 2 - Insert one finger into your vagina and squeeze tight with your vaginal muscles, holding the contraction for a count of ten (if you don't seem able to squeeze tightly enough, use two fingers for now; eventually you will be able to do it with just one).

Step 3 - Relax your vaginal muscles and exhale, but do not remove the finger. Maintain the position and repeat Steps 2 and 3 for a count of 10 to 20: So you will:

  * Insert one finger into your vagina and squeeze tight with your vaginal muscles, holding the contraction for a count to 10. Relax your vaginal muscles and exhale, but do not remove the finger. Repeat this sequence ten times.

* Let's keep it up. Keep the finger in your vagina and squeeze tight with your vaginal muscles, holding the contraction for a count of 20. Relax your vaginal muscles and exhale, but do not remove the finger. Repeat the exercise 15times.

* You are doing well, so let's keep going one more time. This time for a count of 25: Keep the finger into your vagina and squeeze tightly with your vaginal muscles, holding the contraction for a count of 25. Relax your vaginal muscles and exhale, but do not remove the finger. Repeat the exercise 20 times.

NOTE: Perform this exercise slowly. There is no hurry. Synchronize your breathing with your acticns.

EXERCISE CYCLE 3 – SEQUENCE IV

Focus is very important, remember to perform the exercise slowly and take your time.

Step 1 - Remain reclined in bed, or on a cushioned area of the floor, with your legs spread comfortably apart.

Step 2 - Place the tip of one finger just inside the vaginal opening and try, using only your vaginal muscles, to suck the finger inside. The sucking sensation may be almost imperceptible at first, but with practice you will eventually be able to suck your entire finger inside in this manner.

EXERCISE CYCLE 3 – SEQUENCE V

Learning Control

Every day when you are in the shower, insert your middle finger just barely inside the vaginal opening. Squeeze the muscles at the opening, then the muscles just inside, then the muscles further in, and so on, and try to suck the finger deeper inside your vagina. Do not worry if you do not feel any immediate progress. You will soon enough! Practice makes perfect, as they say.

Be sure to practice at least 3 times a week from this point on.

EXERCISE CYCLE 4 – SEQUENCES I TO VI

LEARNING MANIPULATION!

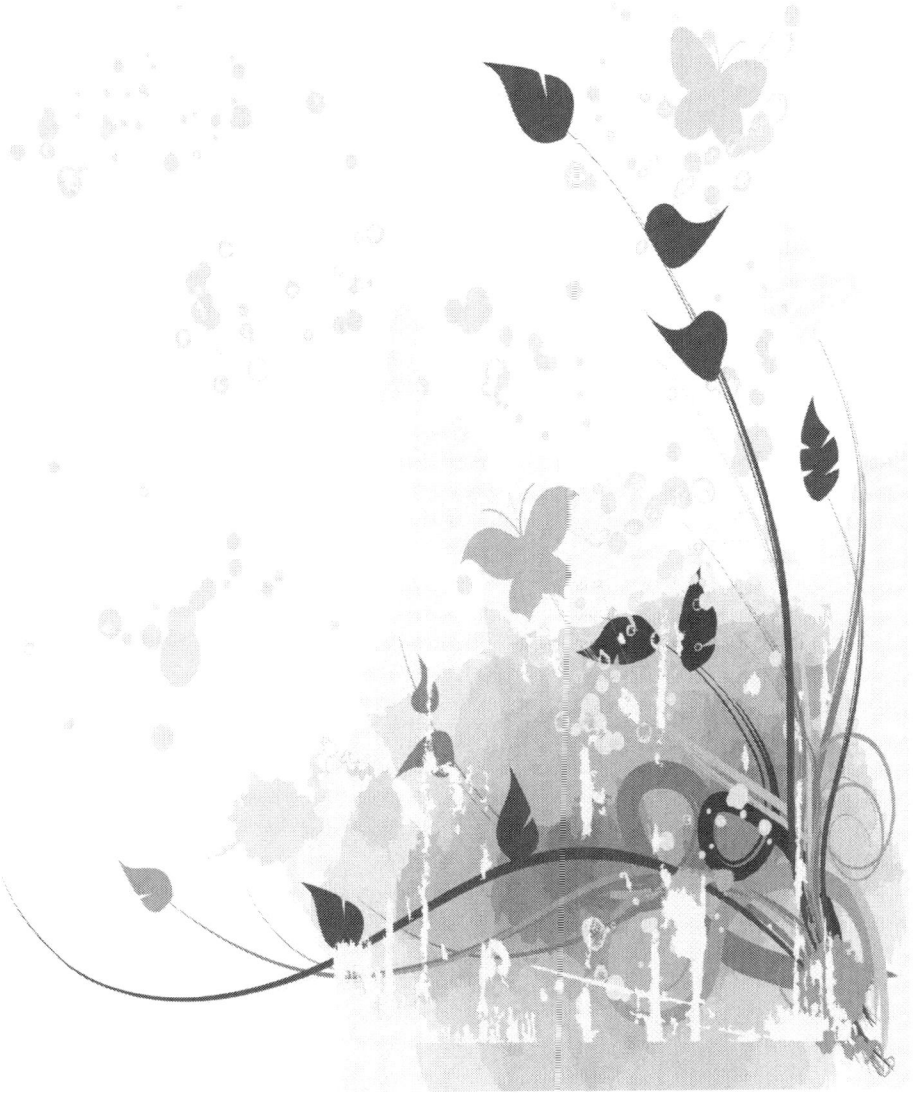

EXERCISE CYCLE 4 - SEQUENCE I

Step 1 - Recline in your bed, or on a cushioned area of the floor, with your legs spread comfortably apart.

Step 2 - Apply gel to the vibrator, insert the tip so that it is barely inside your vagina, and move the vibrator slightly forward, and then slightly backward (not in and out but front to back).

Repeat the movement ten times. Stop and take a minute break.

Let's keep it up. Repeat the exercise. Insert the tip, or keep the vibrator barely inside, move slightly forward, and then slightly backward. This time repeat the movements a total of 15 times. Stop and take another minute break.

You are doing well, so let's keep going one more time. This time, count to 25. Insert the tip, or keep the vibrator barely inside, move slightly forward, and then slightly backward. Repeat the movements a total of 25 times.

NOTE: Perform this exercise slowly. There is no hurry. Synchronize your breathing with your actions.

EXERCISE CYCLE 4 - SEQUENCE II

Step 1 - You should still be reclining in your bed, or on a cushioned area of the floor, with your legs spread comfortably apart.

Step 2 - Apply more gel to the vibrator if necessary (unlikely), and insert it to a depth equal to your middle finger.

Step 3 - Using the muscles inside your vagina, squeeze hard, gripping the vibrator with the vaginal walls for a count of 10.

*Insert it to a depth equal to your middle finger. Using the muscles inside your vagina, squeeze hard, gripping the vibrator with the vaginal walls for a count of 10. Relax, take a minute break.

* Let's keep it up. Repeat the exercise, this time for a count of 15 times, be sure to keep your normal breathing. Take a minute break.

* You are doing well. So, let's keep it going one more time. This time for a count of 25, then relax.

EXERCISE CYCLE 4 - SEQUENCE III

Step 1 - You should still be reclining in bed, or on a cushioned area of the floor, with your legs spread comfortably apart.

Step 2 - Apply more gel to the vibrator if necessary (unlikely), and insert it just inside the vaginal opening.

Step 3 - Beginning with the muscles at the vaginal opening, then using the muscles in the middle of the vaginal canal, and finally using all the vaginal muscles, suck the vibrator into your vagina with three strong contractions. Don't worry if you can't do it at first, or if it takes you more than three contractions. After doing these exercises with the accessories for about five days, you should be able to suck the vibrator fully inside.

* Maintain the position and repeat this sequence 10 times.

* Let's keep it up. Repeat the exercise, this time for a count of 15.

* You are doing well, so let's keep going one more time. This time, count to 25.

EXERCISE CYCLE 4 - SEQUENCE IV

Step 1 - You should still be reclining in bed, or on a cushioned area of the floor, with your legs spread comfortably apart.

Step 2 - Apply more gel to the vibrator if necessary (unlikely), and insert it to a depth equal to the length of your middle finger.

Step 3 - Use the muscles of your vagina to push the vibrator out completely

EXERCISE CYCLE 4 - SEQUENCE V

Step 1 - You should still be reclining in bed, or on a cushioned area of the floor, with your legs spread comfortably apart.

Step 2 - Place the vibrator at the entrance to the vagina - try to suck it into the middle, then expel it out.

Repeat this sequence 25 times

EXERCISE CYCLE 4 – SEQUENCE VI

Step 1 - You should still be reclining in bed, or on a cushioned area of the floor, with your legs spread comfortably apart.

Step 2 - Place the vibrator at the entrance to the vagina, pull the vibrator all the way in – first try to bring it half way, then a little more, then finally all the way in.

Step 3 - Now let's invert the process and – expel the

Repeat this for 15 times.

EXERCISE CYCLE 5 – SEQUENCES I TO IV

Mastering your skills!

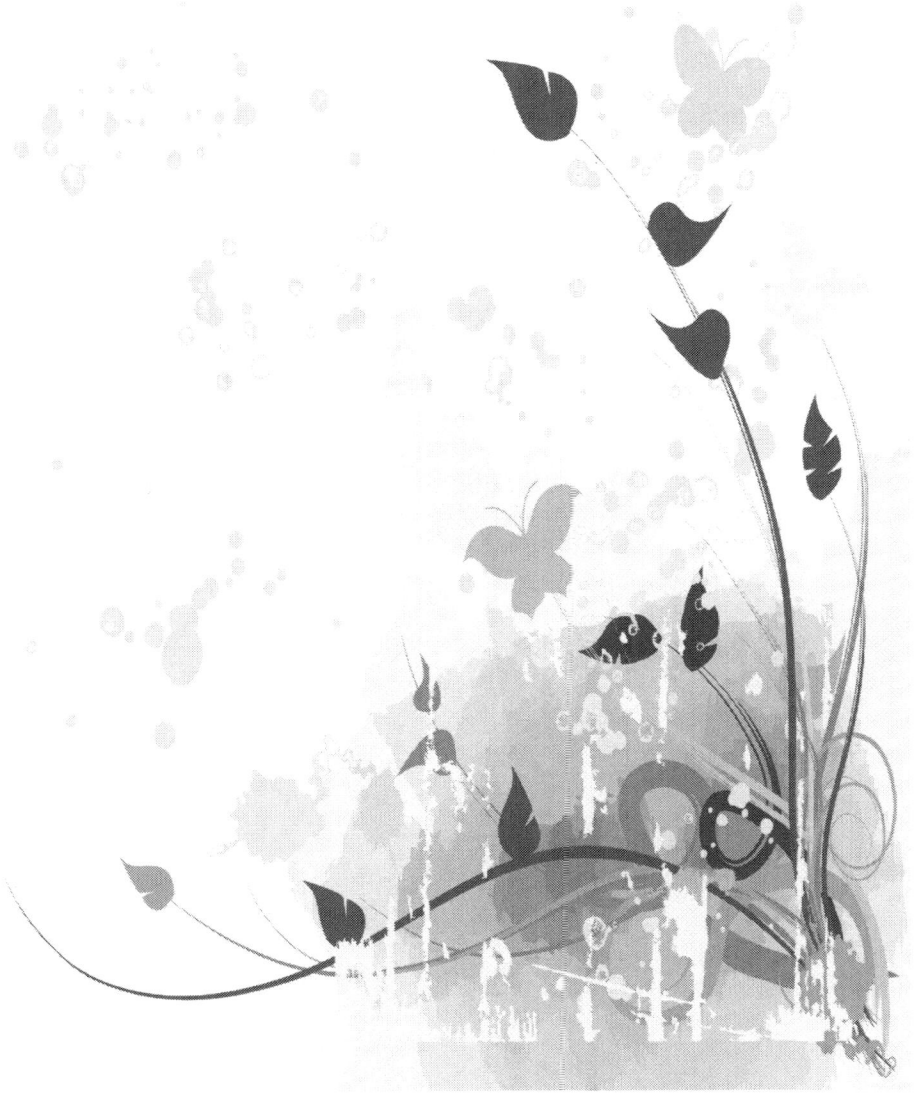

Out and About

Warning: Do not practice any of these exercises while driving as this will hinder your ability to focus on the road, and operating a vehicle while distracted is both unlawful and extremely dangerous.

These are exercises that you can do anywhere - they do not require your full attention. You may do them while walking, in the checkout line at the store, cleaning the house, even sitting on the train.

<u>Step 1</u> - Squeeze, contract and relax the vagina as rapidly as possible for 1 minute.

<u>Step</u> 2 - Move your muscles in a pull and expel motion from *Practicing Control,* in this phase this can be done with our without the accessories.

<u>Step 3</u> - Move your muscles in a twisty motion from **exercise Cycle #6,** perfect for when you are waiting in line. Here, you can do without accessories.

EXERCISE CYCLE 5 – SEQUENCE II - TWISTING

Step 1 - Recline in bed, or on a cushioned area of the floor. Sometimes it is easier when starting out to lie on your side.

Step 2 - Apply gel to the vibrator and insert it into your vagina.

Step 3 - Using only your vaginal muscles (the muscles at the opening will be strongest at first), try to tilt the vibrator sideways—that is, toward one of your hips. This takes serious focus and mental concentration as you try to isolate just the muscles needed to do this.

Step 4 - Now try to tilt just the deepest part of the vibrator to the other side. Although this may take you a while to master, the results are worth it, as the result is that your partner will feel the twisting movements—and it will bring great pleasure to you both.

Note: This exercise takes a lot concentration, so don't forget to focus. As a reference point, you can take a pen, place it between your open hands, slide the upper hand to the right and the lower hand to the left. You will see that the pen twist around.

Step 5 Repeat Step 3 and 4 for 5 minutes. Take a two minute break.

Step 6 - Let's keep going - repeat Steps 3 and 4 for five more minutes

EXERCISE CYCLE 5 – SEQUENCE III - EXPELLING

In this exercise, we want to push the vibrator out with the rings of vaginal muscles, in one fast motion.

Step 1 - Recline in bed, or on a cushioned area of the floor. Sometimes it is easier when starting out to lie on your side.

Step 2 - Apply gel to the vibrator and insert half way into your vagina.

Step 3 - Using only your vaginal muscles (the muscles at the opening will be strongest at first), try to push the vibrator out by using the rings of your vaginal muscles. At first you might think you are squeezing, and that's ok, with practice and time you will be able to tell the difference. This takes serious focus and mental concentration.

* Let's repeat Step 3 a total of 15.times

* You are doing well, so let's keep going. Repeat Step 3, this time for 25 repetitions

EXERCISE CYCLE 5 – SEQUENCE IV - EXTRUDING
(LIKE MILKING A COW)

Step 1 - Recline in a bed, or on a cushioned area of the floor. Sometimes it is easier when starting out to lie on your side.

Step 2 - Apply gel to the vibrator and insert it into your vagina.

 Step 3 - Using only your vaginal muscles (the muscles at the opening will be strongest at first), try to combine the muscular squeeze, lock and suck movements on the vibrator. This takes serious focus and mental concentration as you try to isolate just the muscles needed to do this.

Remember to take your time.

* Let's repeat Step 3 a total of 15.times

* You are doing well, so let's keep going one more time. Repeat step 3, this time for 25 repetitions

EXERCISE CYCLE 6 – SEQUENCES I TO II

PUTTING IT ALL TOGETHER!

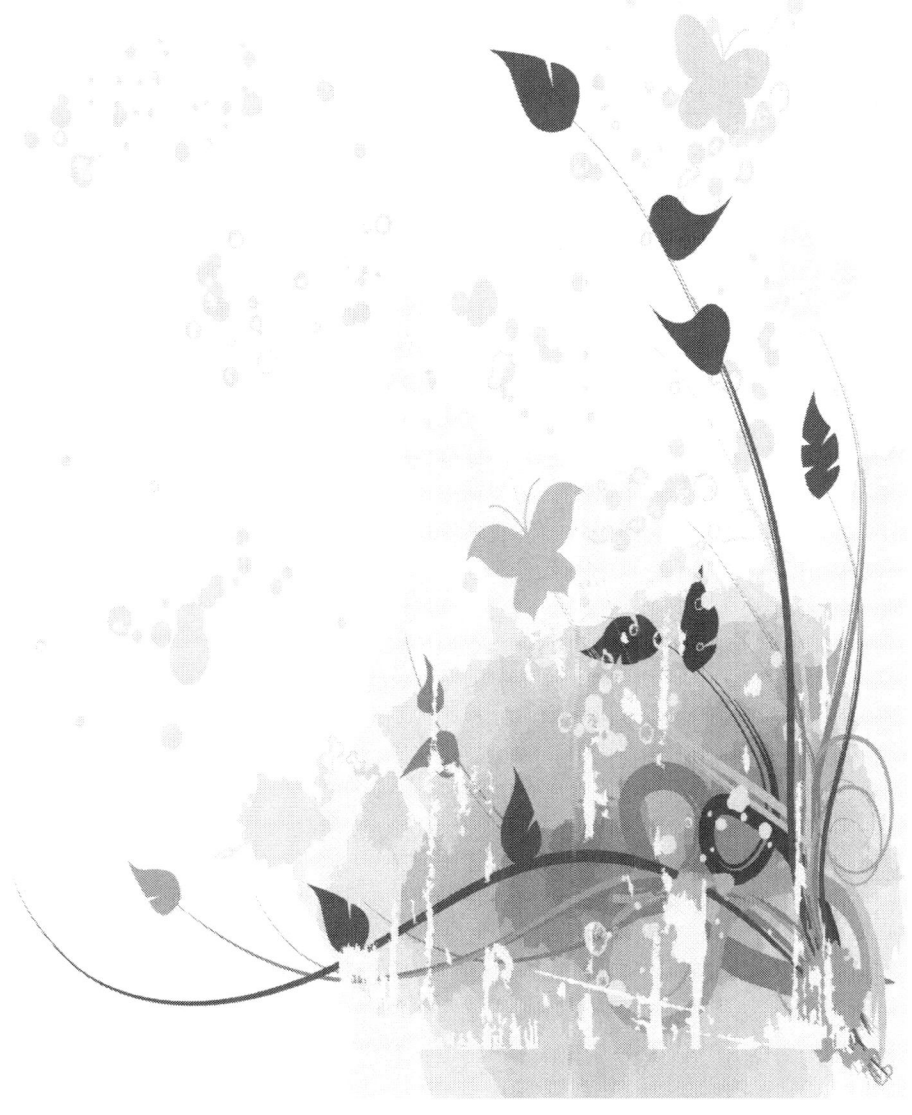

EXERCISE CYCLE 6 – SEQUENCE I

After you have been doing these exercises for several weeks or months, you will be able to use them and combine the following actions into many movements that will enhance the sexual experience:

Step 1 - Lie down, take your towel, vibrator and lubricant, and let's perform the actions below.

1. Pull: suck the vibrator inside the vagina using the pc muscles.
2. Expel: push the vibrator out of the vagina as much as you can using the pc muscles.
3. Lock: pressing the vibrator down with the pc muscles and hold in the vibrator.
4. Grip: Have the head of the vibrator inside the vagina, with the muscles quickly sucking it into the middle and then locking into place.

Repeat each action five times.

EXERCISE CYCLE 6 – SEQUENCE II

Step 1 - Lie down, take your towel, vibrator and lubricant, and let's perform the actions below.

1.   Pulse: contract the vaginal muscles in a fast sequence and with intense rhythm, as if ycu are trying to keep up with panting as you breathe.

2.   Squeeze: pressing the vibrator down with the rings of vaginal muscles.

3.   Extrude "milk-a-cow": combine muscular squeeze, lock, and suck movements on the vibrator.

4.   Twist: move the vaginal muscles side to side when the upper muscle goes to the right and the lower muscle goes to the left.

Repeat each action five times.

EXERCISE CYCLE 7 – SEQUENCES I TO II

POMPOIR WITH A PARTNER!

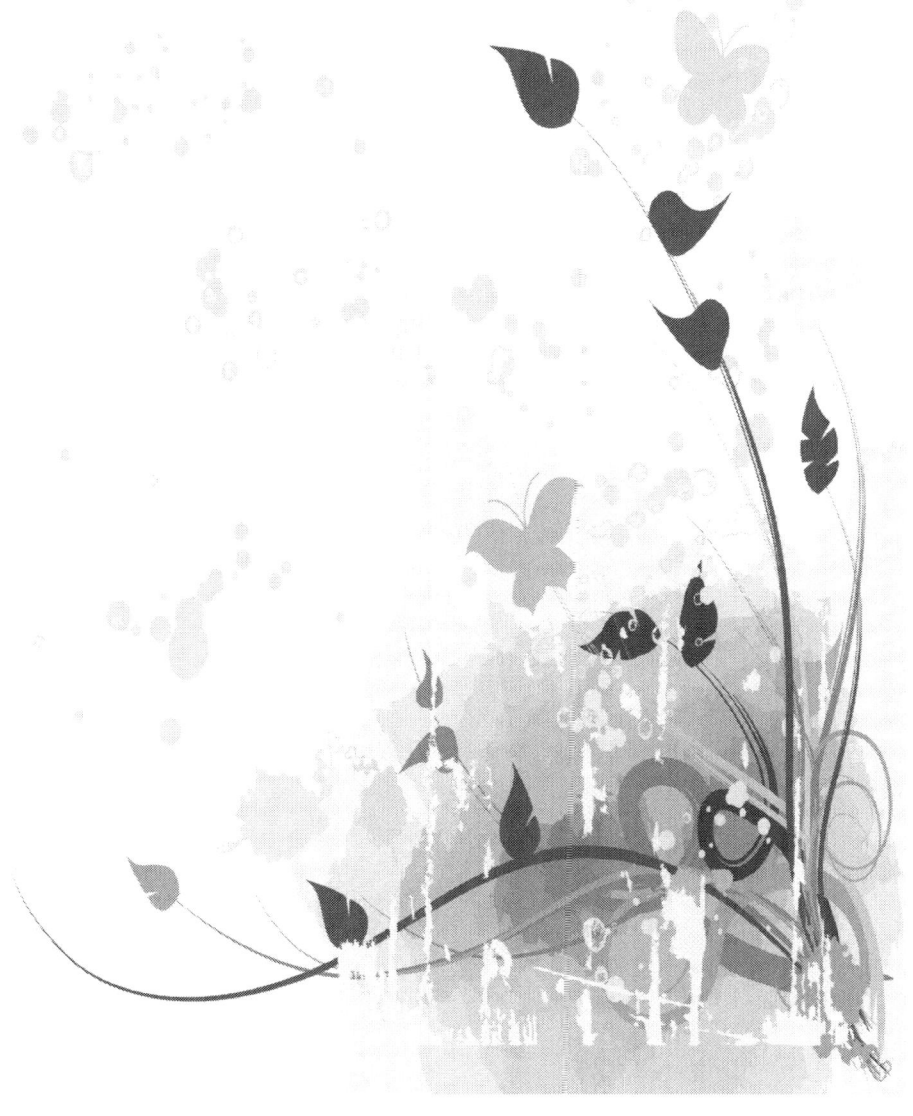

FOR THE WOMEN WHO RAVISH THE WORLD
WITH THE LOST ART OF LOVE

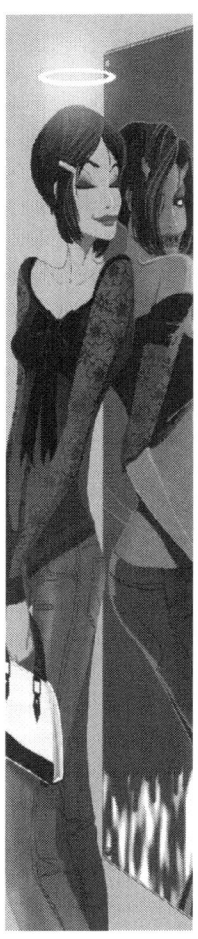

Knowledge is a weapon, don't allow playground bullies to spook you or to discourage you. It is proven that a seductress of the Lovecraft is a goddess, regardless of body type, height or age.

Contrary to the fable, you are now femme vitale, in both personality and technique.

Let your journey remind you that:
« *women who can tap that buried male hunger and provide even a pale reflection of the great sex goddess and a fraction of her* « *everything* » *can name her man.* « Priolau,

That's right ladies, a seductress with advanced sexual skills can keep the man of her choice.

Celebrate your inner seductress.

EXERCISE CYCLE 7 – SEQUENCE I

Step 1 - Assume a position as if you were on top of your partner, sitting on a chair or kneeling on a bed (or if it is easier you can try to do it standing up first)

Step 2 - Apply gel to the vibrator and insert it into your vagina.

Step 3 - Using only your vaginal muscles, try the following actions:

- Suck the vibrator or dildo into the vagina
- Push the vibrator or dildo out of the vagina
- Suck the dildo with your vagina like a pacifier
- Massage the dildo by rippling the vaginal muscles
- Squeeze any or every portion of the dildo
- Pulse your vaginal muscles rapidly
- "Milk" the dildo by squeezing, then sucking
- Lock the dildo inside the vagina
- "Twist" the dildo with sideways movements

❖ Let's repeat this sequence for five minutes, then take a one minute break
❖ You are doing well, so let's repeat it one more time, for another five minutes.

❖ Gradually increase the amount of time you spend on this exercise. As you feel more comfortable, you should try doing this for up to 30minutes.

EXERCISE CYCLE 7 – SEQUENCE II

Now is it time to try these exercises with your partner, and instead of using the vibrator or dildo, you will be using all these fantastic abilities on the penis of your partner, Enjoy!

PERSONAL TRAINING PROGRAM FOR POMPOIR

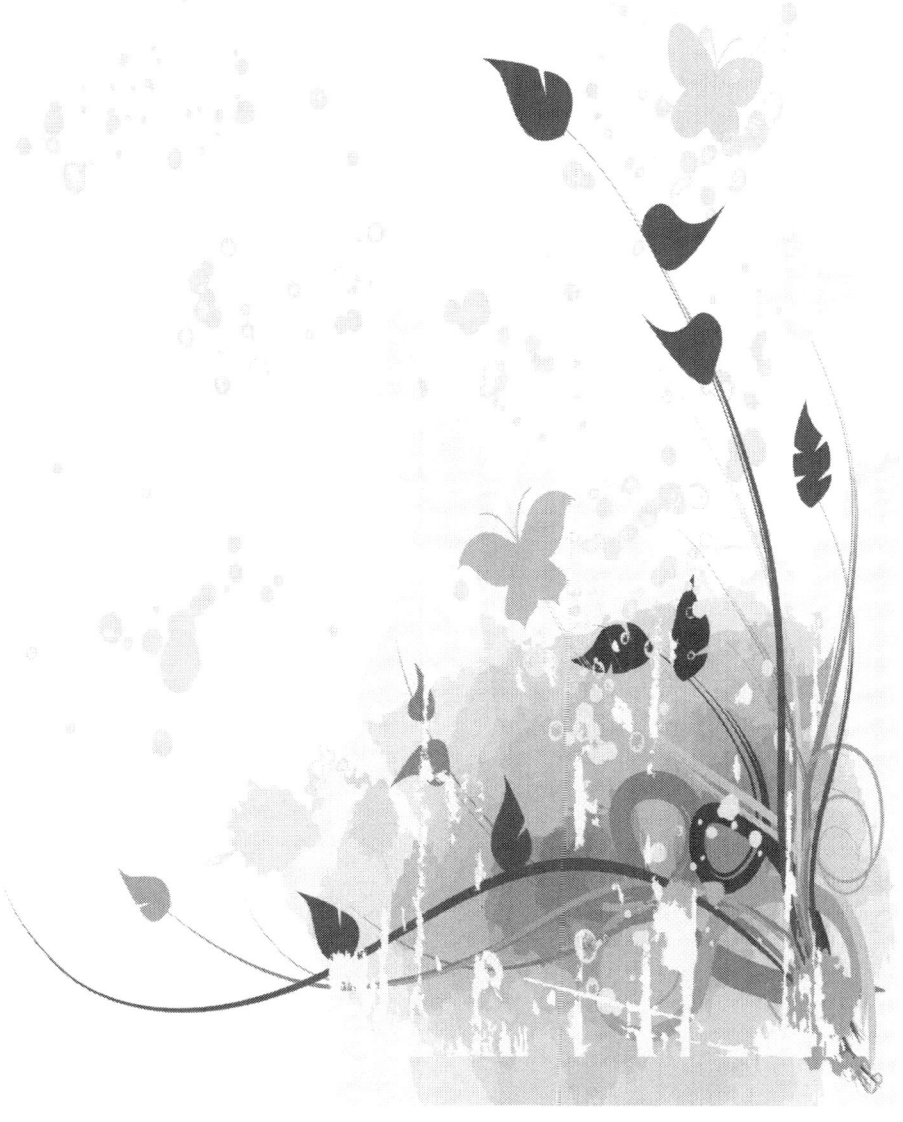

YOUR POMPOIR TRAINING PROGRAM

Note from the Author:

We have found that people have better results, when they start their training right after their period and on Mondays. For those whom no longer have their period, please start on a Monday.

1. "X" - Whenever you see the "X" symbol, it simply means NO training or it indicates the END of the routine for the day.
2. Read the day of the week corresponding with your current training day and follow the sequence asked.
3. Move on from the sequence as soon as you feel comfortable with the exercise and can perform it for the number of repetitions suggested.
4. You will be finished with the routine as soon you get to the "X" task or after the "Stretch."
5. None of the exercises should cause any pain, if you feel any type of pain, stop immediately and consult your doctor.

NO training on Saturdays and Sundays

1st Week's Exercise Routine

Monday	Tuesday	Wednesday	Thursday	Friday
Finding your PC Muscle	Warm up	Warm up	Warm up	Warm up
Learning to Warm up	Exercise Cycle 1- Sequence I to III	Exercise Cycle 1- Sequence I to III	Exercise Cycle 1- Sequence I to III	Exercise Cycle 1- Sequence I to IV
Learning to Stretch	Stretch	Stretch	Stretch	Stretch
Learn the motions Contract, Squeeze, Relax, Push and Pull	X	X	X	X

2nd Week's Exercise Routine

Monday	Tuesday	Wednesday	Thursday	Friday
Warm up	Warm up	Warm up	Warm up	Warm up
Exercise Cycle 1 – Sequence I to IV	Exercise Cycle 1 – Sequence I to IV	Exercise Cycle 1 – Sequence I to IV	Exercise Cycle 1 – Sequence I to IV	Exercise Cycle 1 – Sequence I to IV
Stretch	Stretch	Stretch	Exercise Cycle 2 – Sequence I to II	Exercise Cycle 2 – Sequence I to II
Assignment	Assignment	Assignment	Stretch	Stretch
X	X	X	X	X

94

3rd Week's Exercise Routine

Monday	Tuesday	Wednesday	Thursday	Friday
Warm up	Warm up	Warm up	Warm up	Warm up
Exercise Cycle 1 – Sequence I to IV	Exercise Cycle 1 – Sequence I to	Exercise Cycle 1 – Sequence I to	Exercise Cycle 1 – Sequence I to IV	Exercise Cycle 1 – Sequence I to
Exercise Cycle 2 – Sequence I to II	Exercise Cycle 2 – Sequence I to II	Exercise Cycle 2 – Sequence I to II	Exercise Cycle 2 – Sequence I to II	Exercise Cycle 2 – Sequence I to II
Stretch	Stretch	Stretch	Stretch	Stretch
Assignment	Assignment	Assignment	Assignment	Assignment

4th Week's Exercise Routine

**No exercising on your Period, return during the 5th week (on the first Monday after your period)**

**No exercising on your Period, return during the 5th week (on the first Monday after your period)**

**If you no longer have your period, just take the week off, and return on the following Monday.**

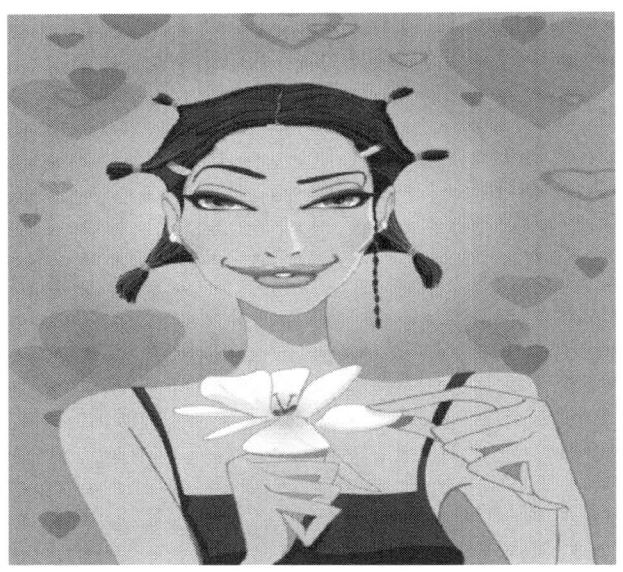

5th Week's Exercise Routine

Monday	Tuesday	Wednesday	Thursday	Friday
Warm up	Warm up	Warm up	Warm up	Warm up
Exercise Cycle 1 – Sequence I to IV	Exercise Cycle 1 – Sequence I to IV	Exercise Cycle 1 – Sequence I to IV	Exercise Cycle 1 – Sequence I to IV	Exercise Cycle 1 – Sequence I to IV
Exercise Cycle 2 – Sequence I to II	Exercise Cycle 2 – Sequence I to II	Exercise Cycle 2 – Sequence I to IV	Exercise Cycle 2 – Sequence I to IV	Exercise Cycle 2 – Sequence I to IV
Stretch	Stretch	Stretch	Stretch	Stretch
Assignment	Assignment	Assignment	Assignment	Assignment

6thWeek's Exercise Routine

Monday	Tuesday	Wednesday	Thursday	Friday
Warm up	Warm up	Warm up	Warm up	Warm up
Exercise Cycle 1 – Sequence I to IV	Exercise Cycle 1 – Sequence I to IV	Exercise Cycle 1 – Sequence I to IV	Exercise Cycle 1 – Sequence I to IV	Exercise Cycle 1 – Sequence I to IV
Exercise Cycle 2 – Sequence I to IV	Exercise Cycle 2 – Sequence I to V	Exercise Cycle 2 – Sequence I to V	Exercise Cycle 2 – Sequence I to VI	Exercise Cycle 2 – Sequence I to VI
Stretch	Stretch	Stretch	Stretch	Stretch
Assignment	Assignment	Assignment	Assignment	Assignment

7th Week's Exercise Routine

Monday	Tuesday	Wednesday	Thursday	Friday
Warm up	Warm up	Warm up	Warm up	Warm up
Exercise Cycle 1 – Sequence I to IV	Exercise Cycle 1 – Sequence I to IV	Exercise Cycle 1 – Sequence I to IV	Exercise Cycle 1 – Sequence I to IV	Exercise Cycle 1 – Sequence I to IV
Exercise Cycle 2 – Sequence I to VII	Exercise Cycle 2 – Sequence I to VIII	Exercise Cycle 2 – Sequence I to VIII	Exercise Cycle 2 Sequence I to IX	Exercise Cycle 2 – Sequence I to IX
Stretch	Stretch	Stretch	Stretch	Stretch
Assignment	Assignment	Assignment	Assignment	Assignment

**No exercising on your Period, return for the 9th week (on the first Monday after your period)**

**If you no longer have your period, just take the week off, and return on the following Monday.**

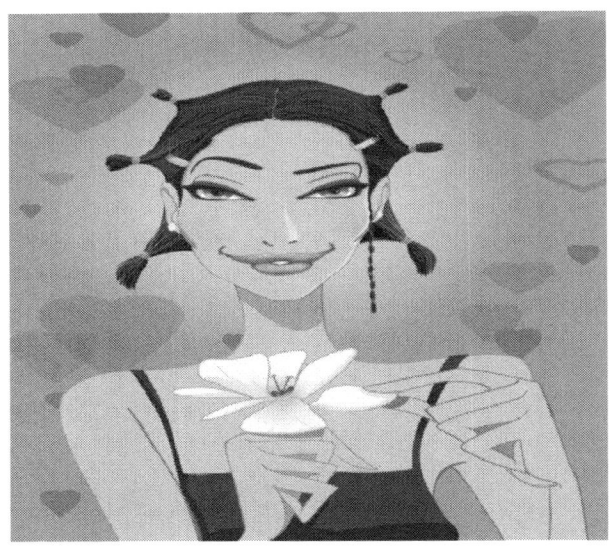

9th Week's Exercise Routine

	Monday	Tuesday	Wednesday	Thursday	Friday
Warm up	Warm up	Warm up	Warm up	Warm up	Warm up
	Exercise Cycle 1 – Sequence I to IV	Exercise Cycle 1 – Sequence I to IV	Exercise Cycle 1 – Sequence I to IV	Exercise Cycle 1 – Sequence I to IV	Exercise Cycle 1 – Sequence I to IV
	Exercise Cycle 2 – Sequence I to IX	Exercise Cycle 2 – Sequence I to IX	Exercise Cycle 2 Sequence I to IX	Exercise Cycle 2 – Sequence I to IX	Exercise Cycle 2 – Sequence I to IX
	Stretch	Stretch	Stretch	Stretch	Stretch
	Assignment	Assignment	Assignment	Assignment	Assignment

101

10th Week's Exercise Routine

Monday	Tuesday	Wednesday	Thursday	Friday
Warm up	Warm up	Warm up	Warm up	Warm up
Exercise Cycle 1 – Sequence	Exercise Cycle 1 – Sequence I to IV	Exercise Cycle 1 – Sequence I to IV	Exercise Cycle 1 – Sequence I to IV	Exercise Cycle 1 – Sequence I to IV
Exercise Cycle 2 – Sequence I to IX	Exercise Cycle 2 – Sequence I to IX	Exercise Cycle 2 – Sequence I to IX	Exercise Cycle 2 – Sequence I to IX	Exercise Cycle 2 – Sequence I to IX
Exercise Cycle 3 – Ben wah Balls - Sequence I	Exercise Cycle 3 – Ben wah Balls - Sequence I	Exercise Cycle 3 – Ben wah Balls - Sequence I	Exercise Cycle 3 – Ben wah Balls - Sequence I	Exercise Cycle 3 – Ben wah Balls - Sequence I

10th Week's Exercise Routine

Stretch	Stretch	Stretch	Stretch	Stretch
Assignment	Assignment	Assignment	Assignment	Assignment
X	X	X	X	X

11th Week's Exercise Routine

	Monday	Tuesday	Wednesday	Thursday	Friday
	Warm up	Warm up	Warm up	Warm up	Warm up
	Exercise Cycle 1 – Sequence	Exercise Cycle 1 – Sequence I to IV	Exercise Cycle 1 – Sequence I to IV	Exercise Cycle 1 – Sequence I to IV	Exercise Cycle 1 – Sequence I to IV
	Exercise Cycle 2 – Sequence I to IX	Exercise Cycle 2 – Sequence I to IX	Exercise Cycle 2 – Sequence I to IX	Exercise Cycle 2 – Sequence I to IX	Exercise Cycle 2 – Sequence I to IX
	Exercise Cycle 3 – Ben wah Balls - Sequence I	Exercise Cycle 3 – Ben wah Balls - Sequence I	Exercise Cycle 3 – Ben wah Balls - Sequence II	Exercise Cycle 3 – Ben wah Balls – Sequence II AND Sequence I	Exercise Cycle 3 – Ben wah Balls – Sequence II AND Sequence I

11th Week's Exercise Routine

Stretch	Assignment	X
Stretch	Assignment	X
Stretch	Assignment	X
Stretch	Assignment	X
Stretch	Assignment	X

12th Week's Exercise Routine

No exercising on your Period, return on the first Monday after your period

If you no longer have your period, just take the week off.

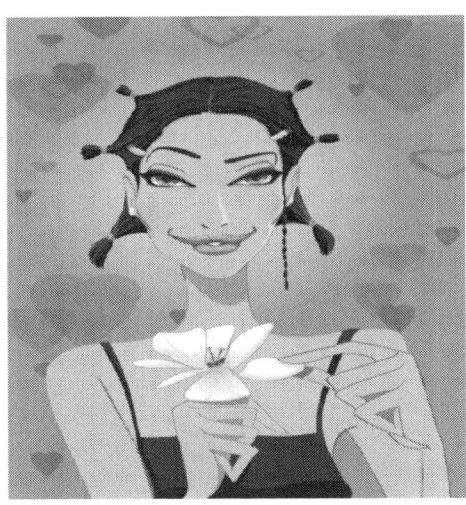

13th Week's Exercise Routine

Building Your Exercise Routine

How to execute your training routine

Because every woman is different, some will have more difficulty training their vaginal muscles than others. Relax, and understand continuous training will ensure success. The average trainee spends from 6 to 9 months mastering the art of Pompoir. For some, it may take longer. Others are fortunate enough to take less time. It all depends on your conditioning, your schedule and your dedication.

Start following the routine step by step. As soon as you master a phase, move on to the next. Try to pick two exercises to practice daily.

The training workout should last for one hour.

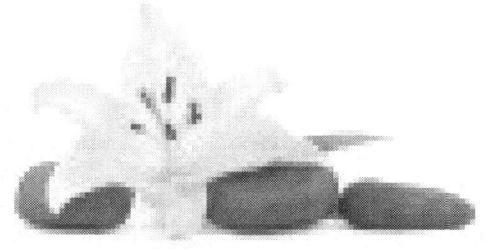

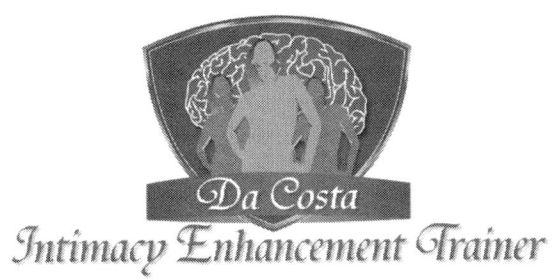

Intimacy Enhancement Trainer

CELEBRATING BEING A WOMAN

www.pompoirbook.com

Made in the USA
San Bernardino, CA
12 June 2015